HOW TO HELP
SOMEONE WITH
AN EATING DISORDER

D1319897

WELBECK
BALANCE

ABOUT THE AUTHOR

Dr Pam Macdonald is a research psychologist, carer coach, and trainer. She is actively involved in supporting carers of people with eating disorders using the New Maudsley Approach, which incorporates the principles of Motivational Interviewing (MI). She also has personal experience of the regular emotional challenges that can impinge upon the functioning of the entire family, as well as friends and significant others, at different points along the recovery path.

When reflecting back on her time caring for a loved one with an eating disorder, she remembers it as a wholly frightening and stressful time. Even after several years, it still evokes strong memories of a long, dismal tunnel littered with countless pitfalls. A major uncertainty was her own role in the process. She desperately craved information on how to react to the situation as well as knowledge and guidance on how to react to the imposter that had invaded family life. She needed to know that she was handling the situation in a way that was conducive to a healthy outcome. In her search for these answers, she stumbled across Professor Janet Treasure's work at the Institute of Psychiatry, King's College, London. Back in 2006, Professor Treasure and her team were working on a skills-based learning intervention for carers of people with eating disorders. Pam joined the project as a PhD student and started work researching the effectiveness of a guided self-help package that offered training and skills to carers.

In 2011, she was awarded her PhD and since then she has worked on a part-time basis with the team on subsequent iterations and development of skills training interventions. She co-edited *The Clinician's Guide to Collaborative Caring in Eating Disorders* (2010)[1] with Professors Janet Treasure and Ulrike Schmidt and has contributed to numerous peer-reviewed papers in the academic literature. She is a passionate advocate of evidence-based research that equips carers with the appropriate information and tools that will help them best support someone through their eating disorder. She is currently based in Edinburgh, Scotland.

HOW TO HELP
SOMEONE WITH
AN EATING DISORDER

A Practical Handbook

Dr Pamela Macdonald

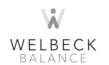

WELBECK
BALANCE

A Trigger Book
Published by Welbeck Balance
An imprint of Welbeck Publishing Group
20 Mortimer Street
London W1T 3JW

First published by Welbeck Balance in 2021

A CIP catalogue record for this book is available from the British Library

ISBN
Trade Paperback – 9781789561975

Typeset by Lapiz Digital Services
Printed in Dubai

10 9 8 7 6 5 4 3 2 1

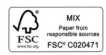

MIX
Paper from
responsible sources
FSC® C020471

Note/Disclaimer

www.welbeckpublishing.com

To Sarah and Malcolm.

CONTENTS

INTRODUCTION

This book has been written to offer you, the carer, practical support, techniques, and guidance to help you support someone who is battling with an eating disorder. Throughout the book, the generic term 'carers' is used whether the person being cared for is a family member, partner, or friend, and the term 'Edi' is used to refer to the person with an eating disorder.

As a carer, you may be eager for as much information as possible to help someone you are close to navigate a path toward recovery, but it is important to remember that you will have your own unique needs too. Parents of a 17-year-old, for example, will face both similar and very different issues and challenges to those parents supporting a son or daughter aged 37. Likewise, partners, siblings, and friends will all have their own questions and conundrums in supporting Edi along the recovery path. This book aims to provide guidance and support to *all* types of carers by tailoring the skills to various contexts and situations.

You may find yourself struggling with mental health issues that stem from your caring role. In addition, although you may feel highly motivated to be part of the recovery process, you may also feel excluded from services or by the person themselves. This may be because Edi is not ready to change and has not yet engaged in treatment, or because health professionals are reluctant to include significant others in the treatment plan, perhaps due to pressure from Edi or because of confidentiality constraints. The consequences can be extremely distressing for all concerned. Throughout this book, there is a strong emphasis on the importance of carers tending to their own needs and health.

As someone supporting a person with an eating disorder you will be aware of the profound impact it has on close others, both through the direct effect of the symptoms and indirectly, by changing the person they know and love. It can feel like Edi has been completely taken over by some monster or gremlin who sits resolutely on their shoulders feeding them misinformation. In my own situation, I screamed, I cried, I bullied, I cajoled, I screamed a bit more, I cried a bit more … but nothing I did seemed to change the situation; it certainly did not result in our daughter eating more. I knew how I was responding was not conducive to her recovery, but I felt that sitting back, ignoring the situation and doing nothing was not an option either. My problem was that I did not know *how* to react. Our beautiful 17-year-old daughter sat beside me with tears running down her cheeks, apologetically telling us she could not possibly touch the salad in front of her as we, her parents, looked on helplessly.

Eating disorder symptoms carry *huge* social and emotional ramifications for families and close others. Whilst symptoms may vary, the impact is frightening, intrusive, antisocial, anxiety-provoking, and frustrating. The physical consequences are alarming and distressing to the onlooker. Normal life disappears, social life and/or any intimacy can evaporate, plans are put on hold, and interactions and communication focused on food increasingly dominate all relationships.

Looking back at that initial period, I did not realize at the time that our own emotional responses to the symptoms may have been inadvertently playing a role in maintaining the problem. Fortunately, the days when blame is placed on the parents' shoulders are well and truly gone, as they should be. This is not about parental blame. I would challenge the most brilliant and competent of psychiatrists or psychologists to sit next to their daughter, son, partner, or friend meal after meal after meal, and not feel anger, frustration, sadness, confusion, despair, and utter desolation at what may seem like a hopeless situation. What carers need is guidance, support, and evidence-based interventions that empower them and give them the confidence that they can play an important role in the recovery process.

THE 'WHY US?' QUESTION

Often the first question carers ask themselves when faced with an eating disorder, is 'Why us?'' The answer to this question is unknown, but what you will learn is that eating disorders develop as a coping response to difficult emotions – and the beliefs that go along with these. Once a pattern of coping by using an eating disorder develops, many different factors, including beliefs about the eating disorder itself, personal habitual thinking styles, and relationships with others and their response to the eating disorder, can all help to keep it going.

There may be fairly 'inbuilt' aspects, such as temperament, personality, or thinking styles, that make someone vulnerable to developing an eating disorder. Research has found, for example, that some people with anorexia nervosa have a tendency to focus on detail rather than seeing the bigger picture. They also find it difficult to be flexible and have a rather polarized thinking style, i.e., unless something is perfect it is 'rubbish' or personally unacceptable. High levels of perfectionism or high expectations of self are also common. There can be a tendency to be hypersensitive in social interactions. The person may, for example, hold the belief that there are negative hidden messages in communication with others, despite there being no such intention on the part of the speaker. As the brain is further starved, these natural inbuilt aspects can become heightened, with the person becoming trapped in a self-destructive cycle.

ABOUT THE APPROACH USED IN THIS BOOK

You have probably come across an abundance of information on eating disorders in your journey so far; some of it helpful, some not so helpful. It can be confusing and overwhelming wading through books, articles, and websites in the quest for information. What is more helpful, however, is information and help based on evidence-based research.

The information and approach used in this book is rooted in the New Maudsley Approach,[2] an evidence-based approach that offers detailed techniques and strategies that aim to improve carers' ability to build continuity of support.

The New Maudsley Method should not be directly compared with the Maudsley Family Therapy programme, also known as Family-Based Treatment or the Maudsley Approach. The latter is a family therapy rooted approach for the treatment of anorexia nervosa devised by Gerald Russell, Christopher Dare, Ivan Eisler, and colleagues at the Maudsley Hospital in London in the 1970s and 80s. Maudsley Family Therapy is an evidence-based approach to the treatment of anorexia nervosa and bulimia nervosa in adolescents. Its efficacy has been supported by empirical research with families. There are three stages: weight restoration, returning control of the eating back to the adolescent, and establishing healthy adolescent identity.

The New Maudsley Approach is not a treatment approach in its own right, but rather an adjunct to treatment for carers and clinicians. The primary aim of the New Maudsley Approach is to reduce stress and empower the family and carers of sufferers. It has a particular focus on older patients and teaches communication, behaviour-change skills, and social support to facilitate change. The New Maudsley Model focuses on lowering anxiety and distress in carers and provides carers with some communication tools to help engage Edi, improve self-esteem, and develop the resilience to embark on change.

Using this approach, my aim is to equip you, the carer, with the skills and knowledge needed to support someone battling with an eating disorder and to help them to break free from the traps that prevent recovery.

HOW TO USE THIS BOOK

In Part 1, we will discuss the nature of the illness itself, how to access help, what to expect upon diagnosis, the impact of the illness on others, common thinking patterns, maintaining and accommodating to the symptoms and the carer's role in recovery. I recommend reading Part 1 in full before moving on to the techniques of Part 2.

In Part 2, we will look at communication approaches using Motivational Interviewing (MI) techniques. There will be numerous examples and case studies throughout that offer the reader ideas on how to tackle and address those difficult and challenging scenarios that frequently arise when living with an eating disorder in one's midst.

Caring for someone with an eating disorder is not for the fainthearted. Some of the skills in the book take professionals years to master so do not pressure yourself to do that. The aim of this book is to equip you with a set of skills and techniques to work and experiment with. You will find the following box placed throughout the book as a reminder to go easy on yourself.

REMEMBER SELF-COMPASSION

The skills and techniques within the New Maudsley Approach represent a steep learning curve. Dip in and dip out of the techniques of Part 2. You are not going to get it right all the time. None of us do ... whether in the New Maudsley Approach or any other part of life! Every mistake is a treasure. Learn from the mistakes, experiment with them and, above all, be kind to yourself. Supporting someone with an eating disorder is not an easy role. Change is difficult for the person you are supporting and changing your responses to them is also extremely challenging.

PART 1

UNDERSTANDING AN EATING DISORDER

1

WHAT IS AN EATING DISORDER?

It can be really difficult to spot an eating disorder. The behaviour of the person who is struggling may slowly change over a period of months, even years and, in the case of younger people, can often be confused with 'normal' growing up or even teenage rebellion. Some behaviours – for example, losing weight or diligently attending the gym under the guise of being 'healthy' or fit – may even be frequently praised. Teenagers may be hero-worshipped for reaching the first sports teams, their prowess on the field being the envy of other parents and their peers. Schools and teachers are naturally impressed and proud of a rising star and, much of the time, the young person's accomplishments and efforts appear to present no justifiable cause for concern.

It took two years for the penny to finally drop that something was not quite right with my daughter. Ironically, I would praise her for her healthy approach to diet and exercise, whilst raising my eyes at my son's lunchbox of crisps and chocolate bars in mock despair! When my daughter became a vegetarian, we put it down as a teenage fad. Looking back, she asked more and more questions about whether certain foods were high in calories. I learned years later that she threw lunchboxes full of healthy pasta salads in the school bin, and 'donated' chocolate chip cookies to friends. During this time, we failed to recognize the early signs of a silent intruder slowly weaving its way through our family unit with the sole intention of strangling everything we held most dear.

SPOTTING THE SIGNS

In *The New Maudsley Skills-Based Training Manual*, Janet Treasure recognizes that the first signs of an eating disorder can be subtle and are often meticulously concealed. She lists some useful pointers that can alert concerned family and friends to the fact that something more serious than dieting is involved.[3] I have replicated these below along with some comments of my own.

POSSIBLE SIGNS OF AN EATING DISORDER
The behaviours listed below should not be used as a definitive checklist. They are more of a guide to the types of behaviour to look out for that can be indicative of the beginnings of an eating

disorder. Any of the behaviours in isolation are not necessarily an indicator, but if you notice several happening or increasing, there may be a cause for concern and it may be time to consult an expert.

- Denial of diet – if someone is actually dieting, they tend to talk about it all the time.
- Change in food rules, e.g., becoming vegetarian, vegan etc.
- Denial of hunger and craving. If someone who hasn't eaten all day says they're not hungry, they're either coming down with a physical illness or there may be something else going on, particularly if there are several other pointers.
- Covering up the weight loss, possibly by wearing baggy clothes. People with eating disorders are also frequently cold, which may be another excuse for wearing large, baggy sweaters.
- Increased interest in food – cooking for others, scouring recipe books, supermarket shelf-gazing, and calorie-counting.
- Claiming to need to eat less than others or only small portions. I have often heard carers complain that they need to lose a few pounds, but daren't eat less than the person that they are supporting.
- Eating slowly with small mouthfuls – tiny nibbles can stretch a mealtime out all evening.

- Avoiding eating with others, e.g., the excuse of having eaten already or eaten elsewhere.
- Behaviour becoming more compulsive and ritualized – cleaning, tidying, organizing, washing, etc. There may be several other comorbid behaviours that accompany the eating behaviours.
- The development of rigid rules about eating, i.e., only certain foods, brands, times of day.
- Becoming socially isolated and low in mood. Previously happy, carefree, and sociable adolescents may turn quiet, introverted, and sullen. Again, this can be mistaken for a teenage phase. If accompanied by several of these behaviours, it could indicate something more serious. Older people may withdraw socially or appear depressed.
- Frequently disappearing to the bathroom during and after meals; the smell of vomit or the excessive use of air fresheners. I would also add drinking excessive amounts of water to this point, which can aid the act of vomiting.
- Self-criticism – dissatisfaction with physical appearance and general achievements, personality and social capabilities; self-deprecating comments such as, 'I'm rubbish', 'I'm such a bitch', 'I'm stupid', 'I'm lazy', 'I'm such a freak', I'm so useless at that'.
- A new or increased exercise routine that is strict, rigid, and gruelling.

- Becoming irritable and angry when confronted about an eating behaviour or exercise routine. To this point, I would also add the 'I'm fine!' mask, usually accompanied by a fixed smile. Other carers I've worked with have also commented on this response. This can be particularly frustrating, especially when you know that the person that you are supporting is anything but 'fine'.

THE DEFINITION OF AN EATING DISORDER

The official definition of an eating disorder – one that is used widely in a professional framework – is that of the American Psychiatric Association who publish the *Diagnostic and Statistical Manual of Mental Disorders 5 (DSM 5)*, which reflects the current state of knowledge and consensus among leaders in the field. The following are the criteria for anorexia nervosa and bulimia nervosa.

Anorexia nervosa

- Restriction of energy intake relative to requirements, leading to a significantly low body weight in the context of age, sex, developmental trajectory, and physical health. Significantly low weight is defined as a weight that is less than minimally normal or, for children and adolescents, less than that minimally expected.

- Intense fear of gaining weight or of becoming fat, or persistent behaviour that interferes with weight gain, even though at a significantly low weight.
- Disturbance in the way in which one's body weight or shape is experienced, undue influence of body weight or shape on self-evaluation, or persistent lack of recognition of the seriousness of the current low body weight.

Sub-types:

1. **Restricting type:** During the last three months, the individual has not engaged in recurrent episodes of binge-eating or purging behaviour (i.e., self-induced vomiting or the misuse of laxatives, diuretics, or enemas). This sub-type describes presentations in which weight loss is accomplished primarily through dieting, fasting, and/or excessive exercise.
2. **Binge-eating/purging type:** During the last three months, the individual has engaged in recurrent episodes of binge-eating, or purging behaviour (i.e., self-induced vomiting or the misuse of laxatives, diuretics, or enemas).

Bulimia nervosa

Recurrent episodes of binge-eating. An episode of binge-eating is characterized by both of the following:

- Eating, in a discrete period of time (e.g., within any two-hour period), an amount of food that is definitely larger than what most individuals would eat in a similar period of time under similar circumstances.

- A sense of lack of control over-eating during the episode (e.g., a feeling that one cannot stop eating or control what or how much one is eating).
- Recurrent inappropriate compensatory behaviours, in order to prevent weight gain, such as self-induced vomiting; misuse of laxatives, diuretics, or other medications; fasting; or excessive exercise.
- The binge-eating and inappropriate compensatory behaviours both occur, on average, at least once a week for three months.
- Self-evaluation is unduly influenced by body shape and weight.
- The disturbance does not occur exclusively during episodes of anorexia nervosa.

Specific type:

1. **Purging type:** During the current episode of bulimia nervosa, the person has regularly engaged in self-induced vomiting or the misuse of laxatives, diuretics, or enemas.
2. **Non-purging type:** During the current episode of bulimia nervosa, the person has used other inappropriate compensatory behaviors, such as fasting or excessive exercise, but has not engaged in self-induced vomiting or the misuse of laxatives, diuretics, or enemas.

Taken from *The Diagnostic and Statistical Manual of Mental Disorders (DSM-5)*[4]

EATING DISORDER MYTHS

One of the most difficult and frustrating challenges for people supporting someone with an eating disorder is working through the myriad of information available and deciding upon the best course of action. By having a sound knowledge of the subject, you will be best placed to help Edi, but Internet searches often lead to that overwhelming feeling of drowning in facts and figures and getting misled by the many myths about eating disorders. Below are some common myths followed by evidence-based answers to help you sort out the fact from the fiction.

> "Eating disorders are thought to be a mixture of biological, psychological, and cultural factors and parental blame only adds to the stress, stigma, and feelings of shame in the family."

MYTH: PARENTS OR MOTHERS ARE TO BLAME

This myth is possibly one of the most unhelpful, at best, and downright dangerous, at worst. Many parents immediately reflect on their role in their daughter or son's eating disorder and feel shame and guilt over their child's diagnosis.

FACT: There is no single cause. Eating disorders are thought to be a mixture of biological, psychological, and cultural factors and parental blame only adds to the stress, stigma, and feelings of shame in the family. The family environment is often the most supportive place to promote and support recovery, but it is vital that parents and carers receive support and guidance in how best to support their child. They can fall easily into certain maladaptive responses due to the sheer stress of having to live alongside an eating disorder.

MYTH: EATING DISORDERS ARE A CHOICE

This myth may use all forms of rationales for how eating disorders develop, especially in teenagers – it is often said they are due to vanity, to the teenager wanting to look like their idol, not wanting to grow up, or simply teenage rebellion.

FACT: Eating disorders relate to deeper issues within the individual and are never ever a personal choice.

MYTH: EATING DISORDERS ONLY HAPPEN TO TEENAGE GIRLS

This myth stems from the fact that eating disorders are most common in teenage girls.

FACT: Eating disorders can occur in people at any age, any gender, any nationality, any religion. They do not discriminate.

MYTH: IN-PATIENT TREATMENT WILL CURE AN EATING DISORDER

FACT: In-patient treatment is sometimes necessary for weight restoration, particularly if the person is at a dangerously low weight, but much of the psychological work is done after discharge. In the UK, current NICE (National Institute for Health and Care Excellence) guidelines recommend that most people with anorexia nervosa be managed on an out-patient basis. This means that the family and close others are very much involved in the recovery process, so it is vital that they are given the necessary guidance and information on how best to support their relative or friend on the recovery path. Edi will require specialist treatment, which can take time. Nevertheless, eating disorders can be overcome and recovery achieved.

MTYH: EATING DISORDERS ARE A PASSING PHASE AND WILL BE GROWN OUT OF

FACT: Eating disorders are a serious mental illness that need specialist care and attention. It is important that people seek help earlier rather than later.

MYTH: THE PERSON IS CURED AS SOON AS THE WEIGHT IS REGAINED

FACT: Once a person's target weight has been achieved, the next goal is maintaining a healthy body and weight without high levels of coercive support and control from other people. Relapse in some shape or form is common and it can take considerable time and work to completely shake off the anorexic gremlin.

You may have come across other myths, which may become clearer to you as you grow in confidence around this subject. Myths can be dangerous and disempowering to all concerned, both the person with the eating disorder as well as close others supporting them.

SEEKING THE RIGHT HELP

One of the more challenging decisions that you will face is knowing when to seek professional help. NICE guidelines recommend that people with eating disorders be managed on an outpatient basis. This places considerable emphasis on family involvement in the recovery process.

Doctors' responses can vary under public health providers (such as the NHS in the UK); some may make a referral with little detail and others may be limited by lack of funding and long waiting lists. Jenny Langley, a colleague on the New Maudsley team and trainer in the New Maudsley Approach, suggests strongly that the more information you can provide in the early stages, the more likely Child and Adolescent Mental Health Services (CAMHS) – or your country's equivalent – are to respond with an assessment.

Adult sufferers may find it more difficult to gain access to treatment for their eating disorder. Services vary by location and carers may be frustrated and hampered in their efforts to encourage someone to seek help, due to lack of motivation on the part of this person or feeling pushed out by the system. As with younger sufferers, the more information that you can present to specialist services, the more likely it is that treatment will be offered.

There are also many ongoing research projects that require adult patients, taking place at any given time. UK Eating Disorder charity BEAT or US organization FEAST may be useful platforms in which to begin your own research (see pages 182 and 184).

> "*You*, as a carer, will be in the best position to pick up on any warning signs, such as changes in behaviour around food, weight, mood, exercise, and body image concerns."

In a private health system, treatment comes with the added financial pressure of being subject to insurance company criteria. The American Psychiatric Association has a chart with guidelines for the level of care appropriate, which you may want to reference when talking with clinicians. This can be found on NEDA's website (see page 184).

We know that early intervention predicts better outcomes and, therefore, it is important to seek and obtain the right help as soon as you possibly can. Although early warning signs can be vague and even appear 'healthy' during the initial stages, e.g., focusing on healthy eating and exercise, whenever these do become apparent, as a carer, you will be in the best position to pick up on any warning signs, such as changes in behaviour around food, weight, mood, exercise, and body image concerns. Consequently, the more detailed information you can present to your doctor, the higher the likelihood of an early diagnosis being made. It is also important that your doctor has experience of eating disorders. Not all doctors do. If this is the case, ask if there is somebody you can talk to who has both knowledge and experience of working with people who have had eating disorders.

Write down your observations in preparation for a doctor's appointment. This will be helpful to your doctor in determining whether to make a referral to a specialist. There are several useful links available that will help you in preparing for an initial appointment. UK eating disorder charity BEAT provides an abundance of useful information to carers and sufferers alike, one of which is a leaflet that provides information to help prepare for an initial consultation with your doctor.

The MARSIPAN summary checklist, created by UK-based specialist clinicians, also provides a list of significant risk factors that warrant urgent assessment, including:

- Recent loss of 1 kg or more for two consecutive weeks.
- Little or no nutrition for over five days.
- Acute food refusal or an intake of fewer than 500 kcals a day for over two days in under-18s.
- Pulse rate below 40.
- Core temperature below 35°C.

In addition, doctors often use the SCOFF questionnaire to assess the possible presence of an eating disorder.[5] This is a simple five-question screening measure that consists of the following questions:

1. Do you make yourself **S**ick because you feel uncomfortably full?
2. Do you worry you have lost **C**ontrol over how much you eat?
3. Have you recently lost more than **O**ne stone in a three-month period?
4. Do you believe yourself to be **F**at when others say you are too thin?

5. Would you say that **F**ood dominates your life?

One point for every 'yes'; a score of ≥2 indicates a likely case of anorexia nervosa or bulimia and warrants a referral.

If you, as a carer, do not feel you are being listened to by your doctor or, indeed, your situation is not being taken seriously, seek a second opinion. The most recent UK Government guidelines from NICE recognize that carers of people with eating disorders should be listened to and supported. Other key points from the guidelines suggest:

1. There should be no delay in referral when an eating disorder is suspected.
2. Physical measurements should never be used as the sole indicators of an eating disorder.
3. There should be clear Care Plans for people admitted for inpatient treatment.
4. People should not be expected to travel long distances for treatment.[6]

Again, you may find it useful to study these guidelines and take detailed notes in preparation for your initial consultation with your doctor.

WHAT TO EXPECT AFTER DIAGNOSIS

"Many carers find the lying, secrecy, and reluctance to be weighed or measured, all characteristics of an eating disorder, very difficult to deal with."

It is beyond the scope of this book to examine the different therapies involved in the treatment of an eating disorder. The treatment plan will be dependent upon many factors – there is no such thing as a 'one size fits all' approach. There are many different pathways and not every type of treatment will work for everyone. On their website, BEAT lists the more common therapies that are offered, which include Cognitive Behavioural Therapy (CBT), Cognitive Analytic Therapy (CAT), Interpersonal Psychotherapy (IPT), Focal Psychodynamic Therapy (FPT), and family interventions that are focused on eating disorders. Your first port of call, however, should be your doctor, who should then refer Edi to a specialist. In working with an eating disorder specialist, the most important aspect is *therapeutic alliance*. It will be beneficial to all if the patient feels they can *connect* with their therapist and the team, in general. This may take a few attempts.

Research has shown that a collaborative care approach can improve the recovery process. As a carer, you are entitled to sufficient information that allows you to provide effective care. Consequently, you should be familiar with the team in charge of the Care Plan, who is providing day-to-day care, including meal support, details of any group sessions or other types of support, information on risk assessment, and review meetings. You should also be a part of any Care Planning meetings and, if possible, receive support on how best to support and communicate with Edi at home. Many carers find the lying, secrecy, and reluctance to be weighed or measured, all characteristics of an eating disorder, very difficult to deal with. If Edi is in treatment, their care team will be monitoring their weight and health on a regular basis. Constant persuading, cajoling, or nagging at home, therefore, may only serve to exacerbate the situation. If, on the other hand, Edi has yet to enter treatment, it will be more beneficial to persuade them to accompany you to the doctor for a physical check-up.

"Using empathy, praise, and affirmations for the efforts of Edi's team members may make the difference between working *with* the team rather than *against* them."

Confidentiality should not be used as an excuse to withhold important information. Most carers respect the need for the person needing help to have personal information kept in the private domain. Carers feel excluded, however, when professionals choose not to listen to information deemed important and potentially useful to the recovery process. If Edi is being treated as an outpatient, the majority of care will fall to the family. Edi may only have one hour a week with the care team, during which time they may choose not to divulge the entire truth. Carers provide continuity of care and so it makes sense to equip them with all the necessary information and guidance required to continue the support outside the therapy room. Likewise, upon discharge from an inpatient unit, the family may be the sole support mechanism. Edi, although physically healthy, will still be psychologically vulnerable. Again, a collaborative approach during the transition period is vital to ensure continuation down the recovery path.

At times, emotions will be fraught, both in carers and the service team. Professionals also suffer from feelings of guilt, exhaustion, and frustration. They may be impacted by limited resources, work pressures, self-esteem issues, and uncertainties. The same preparation and groundwork should be carried out prior to meetings with the care team as you did for your initial consultation with the doctor, i.e. careful planning, prepared questions, and note-taking. The same communication techniques you will be introduced to later in this book (Motivational Interviewing) can be a useful communication style to adopt with the team as well as with Edi. Using empathy, praise, and affirmations for the efforts of the team members may make the difference between working *with* the team rather than *against* them.

MEDICAL RISK

It will be difficult for you to assess medical risk and whether Edi is in danger. Not only that, but non-specialist clinicians who are not used to working with people with eating disorders may also struggle to appreciate the gravity of the situation. If you think Edi's health is at serious risk, then this becomes the number one priority.

Professor Janet Treasure has compiled an assessment of medical risk which can be found at: thenewmaudsleyapproach. co.uk/media/Medical_risk.pdf. This is a useful document to print out and take with you to your doctor or emergency department, highlighting the areas that are of concern to you.

BMI alone is not a satisfactory measure of risk. Edi may have been consulting pro-anorexia sites and these sites produce information designed to deceive and trick people into believing their weight is greater than it actually is. Consequently, a more thorough examination by a medical professional may be required. Other important ways to assess risk include:

- Pulse rate
- Blood pressure
- Temperature
- Muscle strength
- Rate of weight loss
- Blood tests to check any deficiency in essential nutrients[7]

Jenny Langley offers further information on medical risk and advice for support persons in her training manual.[8] Jenny provides a number of pointers to help carers determine whether immediate medical help is required. These are listed below.

You should contact your doctor or get emergency help if Edi:

- Is breathless on lying flat
- Develops a very fast heart rate
- Has a seizure
- Becomes sleepy or twitchy
- Experiences their hands twisting into a spasm (indicates salt imbalance)

Meanwhile, other symptoms that may indicate a medical emergency are:

- Disordered thinking and not making reasonable sense
- Disorientation – not knowing what day it is, where they are or who they are
- Throwing up several times a day
- Fainting or dizzy spells
- Blue hands, feet, lips, and nose
- Puffiness around eyes in the morning and/or swollen ankles in the afternoon
- Collapsing or being too weak to walk
- Difficulty walking upstairs, brushing hair or raising arms for any length of time
- Painful muscle spasms
- Chest pain or difficulty breathing
- Blood in their bowel movements, urine or vomit
- An irregular or very low heartbeat
- Cold or clammy skin indicating a low body temperature of 35°C degrees

2

THE IMPACT ON OTHERS

As well as having a detrimental effect on Edi's health and quality of life, eating disorders impact greatly on close others, who may feel that they're on an emotional rollercoaster. This can have harmful implications for their own physical and mental wellbeing – feelings of frustration, anxiety, helplessness, fear, guilt, and isolation are all common emotions that accompany the task of supporting someone through an eating disorder.

"The eating disorder voice is an expert in spotting any chinks in the armour of those in a supporting role."

'IS IT SOMETHING I HAVE DONE WRONG?'

When an eating disorder emerges in a family setting it is natural to feel an element of guilt, but several decades of research shows little evidence that eating disorders are caused by family. In fact, we know that the family is a valuable resource for supporting someone with an eating disorder. Carers who attend skills workshops, for example, significantly increase the likelihood that the person struggling will be less isolated and have more tools to have a better quality of life and hopefully a smoother road to recovery.

The eating disorder voice, however, is an expert in spotting any chinks in the armour of those in a supporting role. If you are a parent, this might mean you and your partner disagreeing about how much needs to be eaten or what constitutes acceptable behaviour within the home. If you are Edi's partner, you might feel you are persistently nagging at your other half to stop going for that 10-mile run every morning before work. As parents, you might disagree with the care team on a range of issues or just one specific thing. If you are a sibling, you might feel as if you have totally 'had it' with your ill sibling taking up too much of your parents' time. It might be teachers at school or employers giving different messages about the priorities for the person with the eating disorder (exams, work deadlines vs health, for example). It might be the sports, dance, drama, or music coach ignoring health issues in the pursuit of winning or achieving perfection. These things happen in life, and part of the recovery process involves Edi learning to make their own health choices, as well as those around them trusting that they can make the right decision.

PARENTS

The move toward increasing community care for mental illness has meant that families are more involved in providing care to their child. For anybody who has been unfortunate to have lived with an eating disorder in the home, it will come as no surprise to recognize the immense stress and strain that impacts on all aspects of family functioning. What may be less commonly known is that this stress – and the way you respond to the stress and strain – can itself exacerbate the symptoms and generate a number of dysfunctional changes in the family organization and interactions.[9]

> "Encourage all family members to take some 'time out' when the going gets tough. This is as important for brothers and sisters as it is for parents."

Back in 2009, a colleague and I carried out a systematic review of 23 studies that related to the family's relationship with the eating disorder. We summarized the evidence from those studies and looked at levels of carer burden, hostile or critical comments, overprotection (known as 'expressed emotion' in the academic field), and distress in carers, in comparison with carers of people with other psychiatric illnesses. Higher anxiety and depression, burden, and expressed emotion were found in carers of people with eating disorders. This, then, highlights the social repercussions of an eating disorder and how it impacts on the quality of life of *all* family members. The review pointed to the potential benefit of psycho-educating carers to offer information, guidance, and communication techniques. Given the fact that family members suffer from distress, anxiety, and depression, frequently at clinical levels, it would seem reasonable to conclude that they too be included in treatment programmes that offer support and psychoeducational information.[10]

SIBLINGS

Since eating disorders commonly start in the teens and early adulthood, siblings are often involved in many aspects of the illness and recovery process. As a brother or sister, you will experience the eating disorder differently from your parents, first and foremost because you are not in a position of responsibility and can, therefore, feel excluded. You may also be navigating your own tricky adolescent or young adult phase of life and may feel your own needs are being sidelined by those of your ill sibling. Your parents may be in a perpetual state of high anxiety and normal family life may seem to have come to an all too abrupt halt. Nevertheless, your relationship with your siblings, both with and without eating disorders, will extend over a shared lifetime and so strengthening rather than neglecting this bond is very important. You will also offer a unique resource in that you have known your ill sibling before the illness and are also a part of the same peer group. Consequently, you are in an excellent position to help repair the interpersonal disconnection that occurs with an eating disorder.[11]

As a sibling, you may be interested in finding out more about eating disorders and psychoeducational interventions. In *The New Maudsley Skills-Based Training Manual,* there are several worksheets to help siblings support their brother or sister, and get support themselves.[12]

WAYS TO HELP THE WHOLE FAMILY

There are a number of ways in which you as a family can safeguard against the negative effects of living alongside an eating disorder. Some of these include:

- Encourage the continuation of normal pursuits that you engaged in as a family before the eating disorder. Be creative ... if exercise isn't appropriate at that point in time, what other shared activities might work? Quiz nights, bingo games, playing Monopoly?
- Support siblings to engage in non-eating disorder talk with their ill brother or sister. Eating disorders can

dominate family routine and talk. Close that circle – do not allow the eating disorder access into it.

- Keep daily routines such as meals, school attendance, and bedtimes as normal as possible.
- Encourage all family members to take some 'time out' when the going gets tough. This is as important for brothers and sisters as it is for parents.
- Try to be mindful regarding the usefulness of open, calm, and honest communication compared with anger and frustration. Encourage openness in the discussion of feelings.
- Encourage creative problem-solving, e.g., 'That didn't work out so well, how can we do better next time around?'
- Brainstorm new ideas – you may find regular family meetings useful, with a pre-prepared list of meeting 'rules', such as one person talks at a time, listen to each other even although you may not agree with what is being said. Choose a time when everybody is feeling calm and take time out in the event of any emotionally charged situation getting out of hand. These meetings can take place between partners too.
- Look upon any challenging situation that arises as a learning experience. Remember the adage 'every mistake is a treasure' – what can we learn from the times when things don't go so well?
- Promote empathy for each other.

- Remind family members of happier days, using photographs and videos.
- Affirm efforts, goals, achievements and, above all, love for each other!

SPOUSES AND PARTNERS

Although researchers have reported widely on the effects of caregiving of younger people struggling with eating disorders, less is known about the effects of eating disorders and associated caregiving in intimate adult partnerships.[13] Partners have spoken about the trauma of living alongside an eating disorder and how they experience a great sense of loneliness and helplessness, often ending up suffering from depression themselves. As a partner of someone with an eating disorder, it may frequently appear that the person you chose to spend your life with has all but disappeared and that your adult-adult relationship has developed into a carer-patient relationship, or even a parent-child relationship and it can be very difficult getting back on track again. Not only may your partner's physical appearance have changed, but their entire personality, approach to life, and way of relating to you may have become drastically altered. Under normal circumstances, couples may visit marriage guidance counsellors with marital or relationship problems, but when you mix an eating disorder into the scenario, it is difficult to get that type of understanding and empathy unless the counsellor has specialist knowledge in the field.

> "Couples reported that effective non-judgemental listening and communication from both partners was essential for recovery."

Sexual intimacy and relationship problems only add to the difficulties couples living with eating disorders experience. One study, for example, assessed 242 women living with an eating disorder and found that they reported lower sexual desire and activity and increased anxiety about sexual intimacy compared with a control group of women who did not have eating disorders.[14] In the same study, couples identified a variety of effects the eating disorder had on their relationship. In addition to decreased intimacy, there was added stress, tension and conflict, difficulty making plans around food, and lifestyle changes. Couples reported that effective non-judgemental listening and communication from both partners was essential for recovery, as well as the importance of learning coping skills to manage negative emotions.

Support for partners, then, is as important as it is for parents living with an eating disorder and partners too need to have access to interventions that provide tailored specialist knowledge, guidance, and support to their particular situations. As with parents, partners of people with eating disorders benefit from increasing their awareness and knowledge of the illness so that they can provide more effective support.

FRIENDS

As a close friend of someone with an eating disorder, you may experience frustration, concern, and uncertainty as to how to address your friend's apparently irrational behaviour and distorted thought patterns. You may be faced with your ill friend drawing back from the activities and/or hobbies you used to share in the past. They may have lost their usual sense of humour and sense of fun. Furthermore, in friendships, many activities are centred around food and drink – going out to restaurants or cafés – and so, you may have noticed your friend retreating and socially isolating her or himself. Janet Treasure and colleagues draw attention to the fact that friends may be at a loss as to how to react and what to say.[15] Consequently, you may be frightened of saying the wrong thing at the wrong time and it may seem as though your friendship has changed from one of fun and laughter to walking on eggshells or treading across hot coals.

Nevertheless, you can be a valuable resource that links your ill friend to their once healthy life. With understanding and skills in how to address the challenges, which you will learn in this book, you too can be an important resource in the recovery path.

It is clear then that you will have your own individual needs as well as the more generic needs when supporting someone with an eating disorder. Whether you are a parent, a partner, sibling or a close friend, you will need guidance on how best to support this person and help them back on the road to recovery. Case studies will be used later on in the book to represent common scenarios that arise in the various caring roles.

3

HOW EDI THINKS

People with eating disorders tend to share the same thinking styles, many of which are not necessarily problematic under normal circumstances. Traits such as 'attention to detail' or 'focus' can be useful in certain factions of society. For example, when I am in an airplane, I feel grateful and reliant on the attention to detail and focused traits of the air traffic controller guiding us safely down. However, using that same attention to detail in counting grams of sugar or drops of oil in a bid to slowly starve one's body is not so useful. There is no one cause of eating disorders, but it is thought that people with a natural propensity toward attention to detail can be more susceptible to developing an eating disorder if other environmental factors also exist, e.g. perfectionist tendencies, stressful life occurrences.

EFFECTS ON THE BRAIN

To look at thinking styles in a bit more detail, we must first consider the workings of the brain itself. The brain requires a high level of energy to function effectively. It uses about 500 calories a day (or a fifth of the daily calorific input) for all of its many tasks, including perception, thinking, emotional regulation, and memory. In addition to being a major site of energy outlay, the brain is crucial in many aspects of the control of energy intake. Thus, the brain plays a major role in acquiring sources of energy, both for its *own* needs and those of the rest of the body, and so requires a high level of energy to function effectively.

Several functions of the brain are weakened if it is not receiving adequate nutrition, for example:

- **Social cognition:** Understanding how other people tick and deciphering all of life's social signals that help us feel we are part of a wider social group.
- **Emotional regulation:** The ability to buffer ups and down in our mood. Whilst most of us will have experienced some sort of emotional 'meltdown' at different points in our lives, few of us would disagree that these intense emotional responses are conducive to general long-term wellbeing and health.
- **Emotional expression:** People with eating disorders commonly find it difficult to express emotions, difficult or otherwise. Many parents I have worked with have talked about their daughters or sons continually telling

them they're 'fine', with a fixed mask-like expression even though it is obvious that behind the mask, this person is anything but 'fine'. The emotional expression of those around us provides us with a wealth of social information about others. It is as essential to those around us, as it is to ourselves, to be able to interpret and respond to the emotions of others.

- **Decision-making skills:** These are very much impaired in people with anorexia and bulimia. A simple definition of decision-making is the ability or act of choosing one course of action over another. Edi is at the helm of their wellbeing – only they and they alone can make those important decisions that will result in long-term improved physical and mental wellbeing. Consequently, decision-making skills are crucial to recovery.

Brain starvation impacts on the very core being of an individual, causing some aspects of personality to be accentuated or new features to emerge. An increase in compulsive, repetitive, and impulsive behaviours may occur. You may have noticed Edi's increasingly ritualized behaviours, bound by rules and concentrated on small details, particularly relating to food and weight. It is not unusual, for example, for Edi to count grains of rice as if their very life depended upon it. It becomes harder and harder for them to see life's bigger picture beyond this narrow vantage point. Social interactions and communication with others become less rewarding and Edi becomes increasingly withdrawn into their eating disorder world, isolating themself even further from the outside world.

"You may experience sheer frustration and anger when you desperately try to talk with Edi about the pain they appear to be in, to no avail."

Loss of a sense of self and self-esteem makes the regulation of emotions even more challenging and frustration can quickly escalate into anger. Anxiety, dread, fear ... even terror is commonplace, often to the point of panic attacks. For others, the pain of these emotions may be too much to bear and it becomes easier to use their eating disorder to numb painful emotions. To an outsider, Edi can appear emotionally frozen, expressing neither pleasant nor unpleasant emotions. Many carers also experience sheer frustration and anger when they desperately try to talk with the person they are supporting about the pain they appear to be in, to no avail.

For those close to Edi, it appears that the person they have known and loved is lost or transformed because of these deficits in brain function. Parents grieve for the loss of their child. If the person with the illness is their partner, feelings of having lost the source of solace and comfort that intimate relationships provide will surface. You may feel like the possibility of normality ever returning is but a faint dot on the horizon.

HOW CAN YOU RESPOND TO THIS CHANGE IN BRAIN FUNCTION?

In the New Maudsley's carer skills training,[16] carers are encouraged to provide support to shore up this defective self-regulation pattern. Some of the skills and techniques involve the following:

- Becoming highly skilled in listening and maintaining/increasing motivation with regards to the bigger picture of life plans and values in mind.
- Developing high levels of emotional regulation and empathy through a kind, compassionate stance to both the sufferer and their own needs.
- Learning to recognize and accept that we are all products of a complex interaction between our genes and early environmental influences. It is nobody's fault.
- Coaching in the skills of emotional intelligence, encouraging flexibility, and recognizing the bigger picture as opposed to the detail, and in decision-making and planning.

INFORMATION-PROCESSING STYLES

Families frequently want to know why an eating disorder has invaded their family, what has caused it etc. I initially frequently lamented on 'Why us?' Years later, having carried out much research, it dawned on me that the question should have been 'Why not us?' My husband and I both err on the side of attention to detail, perfectionist natures do tend to creep in from time to time. I personally love a routine and feel rather put out if that routine is broken in any way. We know that families are not to blame for eating disorders. However, family members often share similar traits or characteristics that can result in a propensity toward developing an eating disorder.

For those of you who are drawn to evidence-based research, two particular traits evident in people with eating disorders are known in academic terms as 'set-shifting' and 'central coherence'.

Set-shifting: This refers to the ease with which people can alternate between tasks, i.e., how easy it is for them to adapt to change, whether they show flexibility or are a bit more rigid. An example of this would be, say, getting up in the morning having planned to meet a friend for coffee. The friend calls to say that something else has come up and she can no longer meet. Most people would plan another date and carry on with their day. Those with eating disorders tend to rely on routines and can become stressed when those routines change, whether that's in general day-to-day life or particularly associated with food and mealtimes. The disruption to normal life brought about by COVID-19 and lockdown in 2020 was even more challenging for people with eating disorders due to the need for flexibility, both in thought processes and behaviour.

Central coherence: This is being stuck on the detail as opposed to being able to look at the bigger picture or 'not seeing the wood for the trees'. In other words, it's a preoccupation with detail rather than seeing the bigger picture. Examples may include focusing in on the negatives of a situation, instead of standing back and considering other options.

CASE STUDY

One carer told me of a discussion she'd had with her daughter who was suffering from anorexia. Let's call the girl 'Chloe'.

Chloe was feeling miserable, her self-esteem was at an all-time low. After one particularly harrowing conversation, her mum grabbed two pieces of paper, scribbled their names on each one and instructed her daughter to describe herself. Chloe wrote, 'I am Chloe and I'm good at maths.'

When urged to elaborate on herself, she struggled. Mum then took her turn. She wrote down a personality trait of her own with regards to self, personality, talents, strengths, weaknesses etc. This was turned into a turn-taking game and within ten minutes the two pages were covered with a multitude of traits and attributes that make up our unique selves. This was an excellent lesson in encouraging Chloe to see beyond the small detail and not only to see herself in a wider context, but others too. Yes, she was good at maths, and as the exercise progressed, she began to include other attributes – strengths, weaknesses, aspects of her personality, such as 'funny', 'good friend', 'impatient', 'kind', 'loves animals', 'stubborn at times', 'determined' … all those qualities and characteristics that make up the very essence of the human spirit and being.

SHARED PERSONALITY TRAITS

Consequently, shared personality traits and characteristics often run in families of people with eating disorders, in the same way as physical attributes might, such as hair colour. Those with eating disorders frequently show high levels of perfectionism and this same trait can also be found in other family members. A 'drive for thinness' may be transmitted through the family with an emphasis being placed on exercise, healthy eating and a dislike, or even disgust, at being overweight. In his book *The Compassionate Mind*, Professor

Paul Gilbert recognizes that we are all products of a complex interaction between our genetic inheritance and early environmental influences: 'the kind of person we are emerges from the interaction of two major controlling processes that we as individuals have absolutely no control over: our genes and our early environment.'[17] The good news is that Gilbert also suggests that once we fully realize how and why we did not design much of what goes on in our minds, that we can then take responsibility in new ways and learn how to live and work with our own unique mind!

You may find the following activities useful in reflecting upon any shared traits in your own families and a useful discussion point. If you, as a carer, can recognize any shared similarities in traits it may help you to empathize or relate to Edi's difficulties. Give yourself a score on a scale of 1-10 with 10 being 'most of the time' and 1 being 'not applicable to me'. Scores should be used as guides only to allow you to reflect on whether, for example, you tend to be more of a 'bigger picture' or an 'attention to detail' person.

There is no right or wrong answer. The aim of the exercises is to encourage self-reflection, and consider whether Edi may share these traits.

There are boxes at the end of each activity with ideas aimed at encouraging alternative ways of thinking, which you may find useful to try with Edi.

ACTIVITY:
Attention To Details vs Seeing 'the Bigger Picture'

On a scale of 1–10, with 10 being 'most of the time' and 1 being 'not applicable to me', consider the following statements:

- I can have a bit of a blinkered view of things and have difficulty in understanding other perspectives.
- I experience considerable discomfort if things are not as I feel they should be.
- I find it difficult to switch tasks spontaneously.
- I have a tendency to analyse challenges in detail and focus on the negatives.
- If something goes wrong or I feel I've received a negative response from somebody, I kind of dwell on it.
- I sometimes have difficulty following a storyline of a film or a book, but can remember specific details about some aspects. In other words, I can get hung up on the details rather than understanding the gist of a storyline.
- If other people look upset or angry, I assume that it's my fault.
- I get a bit uptight if people don't follow my instructions.

- I often take longer performing tasks than others, due to my attention to detail.
- I have problems with prioritizing and often spend the same amount of time on a task whether it is important or not.
- I have an eye for spotting details that others can miss.

Whilst going through the above points, if any of them resonate with your own personality, ask yourself whether your attention to detail causes any difficulties or problems for you in some situations. 'Attention to detail' is an important attribute in some careers or jobs. If I was due to have surgery, for example, I would hope that 'attention to detail' was very much a major part of my surgeon's personality profile! As carers or supporters of people with eating disorders, it may be useful to role play greater flexibility in some areas of life.

Ways to strengthen the bigger picture

1. Read a newspaper article and summarize it.
2. Watch a TV programme or listen to a radio programme and describe it in three sentences.
3. In five short bullet points, describe what your life looks like, looking back from retirement age.
4. Keep on the lookout for – and note down as many examples as you can of – other people taking a bigger picture other than a detailed approach.
5. Add any other ideas that are relevant to your life.

ACTIVITY:
Level of Flexibility in Everyday Life

On a scale of 1–10, with 10 being 'most of the time' and 1 being 'not applicable to me', discuss the following statements:

- I hate last-minute changes of plans.
- I'm not a great multi-tasker – I much prefer doing one job at a time.
- I don't like new ways of doing things; I don't like change.
- I like things to be in a particular order.
- I like routine.
- I find it difficult to see others' points of view.
- I don't like it when people are not punctual.
- I find it difficult getting back into a job if I have been interrupted.
- I don't like it when other people make changes that affect my plans.

We find degrees of flexibility versus rigidity in all people from all avenues of life. Generally, this is not problematic for the majority of people, but a sudden change of plan, such as a forced change in a daily travel route, may cause considerable trauma to someone battling an eating disorder. Again, as a carer, it may be useful to role play increased flexibility in your own lives. For example, giving a variety of options to Edi will encourage them to make choices – Plan A or Plan B?

Ways to strengthen flexibility

1. Try to make a small change in each domain of your life: relationships, at home, at work.
2. Note down situations that could be described or perceived differently depending on your perspective (e.g. news, opinions).
3. Keep on the lookout for – and note down as many examples as you can spot of – other people being flexible.
4. Select a TV programme you have never watched, switch channel on the spur of the moment, or start listening to the radio.
5. Add any other ideas that are relevant to your life.

ACTIVITY:
Perfectionism and Fear of Making Mistakes

On a scale of 1–10, with 10 being 'most of the time' and 1 being 'not applicable to me', discuss the following statements:

Perfectionism and the impact of excessively high standards on life

- I expect a great deal from myself and others.
- Before I go out, I must look perfect.
- My environment must be tidy, clean, and organized.
- I always have to give my best in all areas of life.
- Even when I have given my best, I am not always satisfied with the outcome because I tend to think I could have done better.
- I can be judgemental with others if I think they have not given their best.
- I check things over and over again to make sure they are perfect.
- If I haven't scored top marks or performed the best, then I feel as if I've failed.

There are many jobs, such as the previously mentioned air traffic controller and surgeon, where high levels of perfectionism are not only expected, but vital. In the case of people with eating disorders, however, they tend to have low self-esteem and can become bogged down with their own self-inflicted demands on themselves, or their perceptions of what other people expect of them. Be aware of this. Adopt the adage 'Every mistake is a treasure' into your own life wherever possible and role play this with Edi.

Ways to work with being 'good enough'

1. Think about your fear of making a mistake. Is it realistic or is it rather out of proportion, maybe a bit like a phobia?
2. Do something spontaneous such as inviting friends over on the spur of the moment rather than for a perfectly planned evening.
3. Halve the amount of time you take to do your hair or put your make-up on.
4. Halve the amount of time you take to carry out a household chore.
5. Add any other ideas that are relevant to your life.

The above exercises are intended to be used as a tool for reflection. We all share similar personality traits, just as we all share physical attributes. It may be useful for those directly related to Edi to reflect on their own personality traits so that they can role-model to Edi that they too can be more flexible, see the bigger picture or make mistakes and the world will still turn.

4

HOW YOU RESPOND

If Edi's eating disorder is impacting you daily, you may find yourselves trying to keep the peace in return for a quiet life. This is very common, especially when you are trying to support someone you love. It is only natural for parents or close others to want to avoid conflict at all costs. I would challenge the most brilliant and competent of clinicians to sit night after night trying to feed and support their anorexic son, daughter, sister, brother, or partner and not experience levels of high emotion in response to what is happening. It is not an easy task. 'Walking on eggshells' is a term I hear frequently when talking with carers.

"As parents, we care for our children from the cradle and it can be difficult for us to realize that our nurturing actions could actually be *enabling* the eating disorder."

Being accommodating and enabling are very natural responses to caring for somebody who is sick. As parents, we care for our children from the cradle and it can be difficult for us to realize that our nurturing actions could actually be *enabling* the eating disorder. Parents, or perhaps partners, can find themselves covering up or removing negative consequences of Edi's behaviour – for example, by cleaning the bathroom or kitchen after a binge. They can become prisoners themselves to eating disorder food rules or safety behaviours, which may involve excessive exercise, vomiting, body-checking, and fasting, or restricting as well as obsessive compulsive behaviours such as reassurance-seeking, counting, checking, and control. Sufferers may also appear to control, compete, compare, or attune themselves with other family members in terms of what and how much they eat or exercise. Again, this behaviour is tolerated, with family members accommodating and/or enabling the symptoms in an effort to restore a calmer environment for all.[18]

Of course, it may not always be possible to 'keep the peace' and there will be hostile or critical confrontations. Unfortunately, these confrontations can make Edi feel alienated and they may retreat into the comfort of their eating disorder behaviour even more. You may well regret reacting a certain way after the event, but you are human and this is a highly emotional situation.

These types of reactions can cause ruptures in the family. If the needs of other family members are neglected or if two carers exhibit different caring styles or responses to the illness, it can cause hostility and resentment from all concerned.

'HIGH EXPRESSED EMOTION'

Given this, unsurprisingly, the research points to the potential impact of carers' own responses to eating disorder behaviours and symptoms – for example, the way in which close others respond to the symptoms of an eating disorder may have a considerable impact on the course of the illness. According to a prominent paper on the maintenance factors of an eating disorder, Professors Ulrike Schmidt and Janet Treasure, two world-renowned psychiatrists in the field of eating disorders, found that the reaction of close others, particularly family members, can adversely affect outcome. If, for example, close others respond with even mild critical or hostile comments, this can adversely affect the outcome. Alternatively, wrapping someone up in cotton wool, in an effort to protect them, can also have an adverse effect.[19] Both the aforementioned emotional and behavioural responses are referred to in psychiatry as 'high expressed emotion' and they have been found to be key factors that predict relapse across all psychiatric disorders, particularly in anorexia nervosa.[20]

The good news is that carer interventions have been developed that focus on more adaptive communication approaches to eating disorder symptoms. Carers are offered alternative communication and behavioural responses that can lower high expressed emotion. It is important that you are provided with the information, skills, and techniques that will equip you to best deal with the symptoms and feel a sense of empowerment within yourself.

> "I had no idea how I should react. Should I ignore it? Should I come down even harder? Should I guilt trip?"

Chapters 6 and 7 of this book will explore an alternative way of communicating with the person that you are supporting.

You may be surprised at how many accommodating and enabling behaviours you use on a daily basis. The Accommodation and Enabling Scale is a useful gauge to help carers reflect on whether they are being pulled into responding in such a way.[21] If you want to assess yourself, turn to the questionnaire on page 169.

WHAT'S YOUR RESPONSE STYLE?

On a personal note, I had no idea how to respond to the symptoms when the eating disorder invaded our family. I knew I was not handling it in the most helpful manner, but my problem was that I had no idea how I should react. Should I ignore it? Should I come down even harder? Should I guilt trip? Should I spend my every waking moment attending to the eating disorder and its needs? At that time, there did not seem to be anybody around who could answer these questions or point me in any direction with regards to guidance.

One of the first skills I personally found helpful from the New Maudsley Approach is its series of animal metaphors.[22] These were devised to help carers reflect on their own responses to the symptoms and are a lighthearted way to work with some difficult emotional and behavioural responses. Some 'animals' might be your own natural default way of coping with stress or part of your natural temperament. Some carers I have worked with lament on how they have gone through the whole menagerie in their responses to the eating disorder. This is common. One day there will be tears, other days, anger and frustration. We may choose to ignore it all just to keep the peace and we will also choose to protect our relative or friend by seemingly wrapping them up in cotton wool to avoid further distress. Personally, I was predominantly a rhinoceros, but I did have many kangaroo and jellyfish moments thrown in for good measure!

There is no such thing as a wrong animal response. There will be times when a behaviour is useful: to protect, to be decisive, to ignore, to be upset. You need to learn to judge what works, when. If something is working, do more of it; if something is not working, review, reflect, and try something else. Sometimes it might be that you role-model to the person with the eating disorder that they are only human and, at times, you need to shout, cry, hide away, and overprotect for their own sanity. As the recovery journey progresses, you may find that different responses come more naturally.

CAUTION
When medical risk is high (see page 21), it is of course entirely appropriate for you to step in and take on the responsibility of a duty of care that society expects when a person cannot do it themselves.

The following carer styles are divided into emotional and behavioural approaches.

EMOTIONAL RESPONSES
The jellyfish: Some carers find it difficult to regulate their own intense emotional responses to the eating disorder. You may

find yourself becoming highly distressed, angry, or both. When emotions are running high, it will be difficult to think straight or to steer a clear path. Also, just like the real jellyfish, intense anger and anxiety can wield a poisonous sting in that Edi mirrors similar uncontrolled emotions, which unfortunately, serves to strengthen the eating disorder's hold. These high emotions escalate causing tears, tempers, and sleepless nights, and are exhausting for everybody.

The ostrich: When you find it really tough to cope with living daily life alongside an eating disorder, you may have some 'ostrich' moments. Amidst the chaos and confusion, there can be a natural tendency to stick your head in the sand. You may have found this approach to be a tried-and-tested method of dealing with difficult situations in the past, but Edi can misinterpret it as uncaring or disinterested, and feel unloved. Self-esteem is sapped away. Additionally, hiding your emotions sets an unhelpful example for Edi to follow. It is more conducive to recovery when you set an example of emotional honesty and openness, whilst spreading the message that having controlled emotions is normal and acceptable human behaviour. This will then hopefully help Edi in coming to terms with their own difficulties with emotional expression. Living alongside others who are able to communicate their feelings with words will set a good example to Edi to change their own way of expressing emotions, which is currently through food.

The St Bernard dog: The optimal emotional response is one of calmness, warmth, and compassion. This involves accepting and processing the pain resulting from what is lost through the eating disorder and developing reserves of kindness, gentleness, and love. The St Bernard instils hope in Edi that they can change, that there is a future full of possibility beyond the eating disorder. The St Bernard responds consistently and is calm, unfailing, reliable, and dependable in all circumstances.

BEHAVIOURAL RESPONSES

The kangaroo: You may also find yourself doing everything in your power to protect Edi. You may feel that you are forced to take over all aspects of Edi's life, to treat them with kid gloves and keep them safe in your kangaroo pouch in an effort to avoid any upset or stress. The disadvantage of this 'kangaroo' response is that Edi does not learn how to approach and master life's challenges. We all learn through mistakes and our confidence is bolstered when we figure out our own answers to problems. Kangaroo responses do not allow this to happen.

"The more you argue for change, the more resistance you are likely to face, giving Edi the opportunity to practise arguments for the status quo."

The rhinoceros: If you often attempt to persuade and convince, usually by argument and confrontation, these are known as 'rhinoceros' behaviours. Your response may be due to a demanding home environment that causes considerable stress, exhaustion, and frustration or it could be your own natural default position of problem-solving. The downside is that even when Edi follows the rules or commands, their confidence to continue to do so without assistance is not developed. The more common response to a rhino command is usually to shout back louder with an even stronger eating disorder voice. However, the more you argue for change, the more resistance you are likely to face, giving Edi the opportunity to practise arguments for the status quo. This allows the eating disorder to bury itself even deeper into the person's psyche. A key skill is to allow Edi the opportunity to present their own arguments as to why change is preferable.

The terrier: I'm sure most parents of teenagers will recognize the terrier type of response, one of persistently cajoling and nagging, even *without* an eating disorder. However, nagging a person with an eating disorder is more likely to be perceived as irritating white noise and lead to hidden negative counteracting behaviours. Motives are misunderstood and everyone's morale is sapped. The eating disorder itself also resembles a terrier, constantly criticizing Edi, sitting on their shoulder and telling them, 'You're not good enough!', 'You need to try harder!', or 'You're weak!'. Role-modelling active listening and reflection with compassion and sensitivity directed to the positive will support and encourage Edi to challenge this eating disorder voice.

The dolphin: An optimal way of helping someone with an eating disorder is to gently nudge them along. We use the analogy of imagining this person at sea. The eating disorder identity is their life vest. They are unwilling to give up the safety of this life vest, preferring instead to hang on to their perceived safety of the illness. You are their dolphin, nudging them to safety, at times swimming ahead, leading the way, showing them new vistas; at other times swimming alongside with encouragement, or even quietly swimming behind, showing trust that they will, one day, return to swimming alone with confidence.

Do any of the animal styles resonate with you as a carer, or as a partner, sibling, or friend? You may be interested to know that professionals in clinical settings also find themselves adopting a particular animal style of responding to their patients.

Many carers I have worked with throughout the years have found the animal analogies helpful and a simpler way of communicating caring styles and natural responses to difficult situations. Some carers, however, are not so keen and this is okay too. Sometimes, you may feel a rhinoceros response is very much required – for example, when there is high medical risk (see page 21). We always take the stance of 'whatever works best for you is the way to go'. You are the expert. These are ideas and approaches that may or may not be helpful in your situations. In our family, the animal analogies provided a lighthearted tool that addressed potentially problematic responses. My daughter, for example, would often chastize me for sticking my rhino horn right through the dolphin's blowhole. Once emotions had subsided, it gave us the opportunity to revisit the emotional meltdown and discuss how we could handle the situation in a more adaptive manner the next time.

PART 2

HOW YOU CAN HELP

5

YOUR ROLE IN RECOVERY

The burning question for most carers of people with eating disorders is *what* you can actually do. *How* can you best support someone with an eating disorder? How should you respond and/or behave? What is helpful support, and what is unhelpful?

STAGES OF CHANGE

One important aspect to consider is the stage of illness Edi is in, and to do this we need to turn to the field of Health Psychology and Models of Health Change. In its simplest form, these models are based on the fact that most people have behaviours that they know are unhelpful or situations where they would like to see change. Many people also experience a certain degree of ambivalence as to whether they want or, indeed, would be able to change those situations or behaviours. The basic premise of the Transtheoretical Model of Change is that there are several changes that the person will go through with the target behaviour.[23] They may go round this circle several times before they finally break free. However, every time they do go round, they pick up and utilize strengths from previous times and eventually these gains enable them to completely break free from it.

Model of Health Change

Above: *The Transtheoretical Model of Health Change:* Prochaska and DiClemente[24]

Let's look at these stages in greater detail.

THE PRECONTEMPLATION STAGE

This stage is when the individual has no intent to change behaviour in the near future. Pre-contemplators are characterized as resistant and unmotivated and unreceptive to any information, discussion, or thought with regards to targeted health behaviour.

"Edi may go round this circle several times before they finally break free. However, they pick up and utilize strengths from previous times and eventually these gains enable them to completely break free from it."

Example: You have started to notice Edi counting calories and obsessing about what you are putting into the meals you cook. There may be other indications such as low mood and obsessive compulsions. However, when raised, Edi denies there is anything wrong. Even if you do manage to get her to a doctor or into therapy, Edi may continue to dig her heels in and insist that there is nothing wrong, whilst asking you time and time again why you are making such a big deal of this. Edi may try and pin the blame on you for being too paranoid, overanxious, overbearing etc. This will be an extremely frustrating time for all.

THE CONTEMPLATION STAGE

This is the stage when there is recognition of the problem, initial consideration of behaviour change and information-gathering about possible solutions and actions. People are generally ambivalent during this stage, moving back and forth between the possibility of change and keeping the status quo.

Example: Edi may begin to complain about certain aspects of their life, hinting that there might be a problem. They may feel cold all the time and lack the energy and concentration from healthier times. However, this can swing back and forth. They may talk about seeking help one minute and the next minute deny there is anything wrong at all.

THE PREPARATION STAGE

This involves introspection about the decision, reaffirmation of the need and desire to change behaviour, and completion of final pre-action steps.

Example: Edi is becoming increasingly fed up. They begin to reflect on previous times of their life without the eating disorder and start to take an interest in some of the leaflets and information you provided. They may ask for your support in finding help.

ACTION STAGE

During this stage the individual makes overt, perceptible lifestyle modifications.

Example: Lifestyle modifications are put into place, appointments made, meal plans drawn up. Edi becomes more open and honest about their illness and potential recovery path.

THE MAINTENANCE STAGE

This stage is characterized by a consolidation of the behaviours initiated during the action stage and will either be followed by 'termination' or 'relapse'.

Example: There may be several relapse periods. However, Edi will be able to draw on the skills from earlier successful efforts at beating the illness, using this knowledge and experience to fight a stronger battle during subsequent attempts.

THE CARER'S ROLE

If we consider the above model, let's now look closer at your role as the carer. Using my own example, I screamed, I bargained, I tried to talk my daughter through the reasons to change (her future, going off to university, her health, holidays with her friends etc.). The problem was that I was always in the 'Action' phase whilst she whirled around that circle. This is not only a problem with carers at home. Clinicians working in professional settings also encounter this challenge of being in 'Action' whilst their patients are spinning around that circle.

"Try not to reason logically with the eating disorder – this does not work. At worst, it strengthens Edi's beliefs and arguments for sticking with the status quo."

So how can people best support someone with an eating disorder in the same framework? There are various strategies and techniques that can be applied throughout the various stages.

PRECONTEMPLATION

During this stage, it is not that Edi can't see the solution – they cannot see the problem. When precontemplators enter therapy, they often do so because of pressure from others. They may even demonstrate change as long as the pressure is on. Once the pressure is off, however, they often quickly return to their old ways. Precontemplators can, at times, want to change but this seems to be quite different from intending to or seriously considering change, say, in the next six months. For example, a partner's plea urging the person that they are supporting not to run 10K a day will be met with derision. Why should anybody in their right mind want to stop them from pursuing a healthy activity? Resistance to recognizing or modifying a problem is the hallmark of precontemplation. Here are some DOs and DON'Ts of precontemplation:

DO

- Try to connect with Edi by talking about any non-eating disorder subject, such as current affairs.
- Spend time doing things you both enjoy – neutral activities that don't involve any food talk, eating, or exercise will possibly generate the best responses.
- Try to be non-judgemental and remain warm and accepting, yet have firm personal boundaries and limits.
- Try not to reason logically with the eating disorder – this does not work. At worse, it strengthens Edi's beliefs and arguments for sticking with the status quo.
- Try to give other family members time – siblings, children, partners also have needs. Role-model to Edi that they may allow the eating disorder to destroy their life, but you will not allow it to destroy the other members of the family.
- Try not to get into endless cycles of reassurance, as this does not actually help the sufferer (see page 149).
- Try to understand why staying in the eating disorder is so important to Edi. There must be some benefits, otherwise why stick with it? Although it may go against the grain, try to discuss the pros and cons of change with Edi.

- Look after yourself. Maintain your own interests and life and encourage the rest of the family to do the same. If Edi wants to join in, encourage it.
- Reflect on what you are seeing with regards to Edi's health. This should be done in a non-judgemental manner and not in an accusatory tone. Give feedback about what you see, connecting the eating disorder and its consequences (e.g., feeling cold, tired, lacking concentration, withdrawing socially, looking unhappy etc.).
- Provide education – leaflets, books, self-help, helpful online links and websites, treatment, and outcomes.
- Find medical and nutritional information (e.g., building bones and the nutrition they need).
- Separate the person from the eating disorder, which you could call 'the anorexia minx', 'gremlin' etc. Some sufferers do not take kindly to separating the eating disorder from their sense of self. It can be important for you, however, to remember Edi before the eating disorder took over and that this current behaviour and emotional maelstrom belongs to the illness and not the person.
- Remember to praise the non-eating disorder activities. Praise the process, not the outcome, the fact that it must be difficult for them and that they're doing really well, fighting back hard etc.
- Notice and affirm any small, positive changes.

"Remember that conflict and high emotional stress can make it harder for Edi to talk about their worries and concerns."

DON'T

- Remember at the precontemplation stage, any arguments for change from you will result in even more resistance from Edi. It will also give them the opportunity to rehearse stronger arguments to stay the same. Instead of giving direct advice or suggestions, use a more indirect context. For example, you could say, 'Other people tell me …' , 'Books say …', 'Have you noticed that …?', 'Can I share with you … ?'
- Remember that conflict and high emotional stress can make it harder for Edi to talk about their worries and concerns.
- Do not argue with logic – this rarely, if ever, works with an eating disorder.
- Do not give advice or try to 'fix' Edi.
- Do not use 'why' questions. These can come across as accusatory and will be met with an even stronger wall of resistance.

CONTEMPLATION

This is the stage when people are aware that a problem exists and are seriously thinking about overcoming it, but have not yet made a commitment to take action. They may gently touch on reasons why their current behaviour is less than helpful to them and this is what I used to refer to as a 'golden opportunity moment'. It gives you the chance to encourage the person to further explore the negative consequences. Sufferers can remain in the contemplation stage for long periods, indicating that they perhaps want to experiment with change, but are not quite ready yet. Strategies for this stage include:

- Help Edi to generate a list of pros and cons of change.
- Keep making a connection between the eating disorder and its consequences. For example, 'On the one hand you're talking about our trip to Australia next year, yet this situation you're in is wreaking havoc with lots of your future plans. How do you think it'll go if the eating disorder comes along with us?'
- Explore difficulties in change. Change is tough or challenging for most of us. What are some of the difficulties Edi may envisage? What alternative strategies can they explore? What support would they need?
- Discuss possible plans of action.

- Again, as with precontemplators, encourage any talk about the negative consequences of the eating disorder as and when it occurs.
- Emphasize autonomy, i.e., focus on the choices Edi may have, rather than giving advice. Dialogue that raises arguments for change has greater strength when it comes from the person themself.

PREPARATION

This stage combines intention and behaviour. Individuals in this stage usually intend to take imminent action or have unsuccessfully taken action in the past year. Strategies for this stage include:

- Ask Edi if they would like to include you in their plan in some way. Reiterate that you are there for them in terms of support.
- What do they find unhelpful?
- What do they find helpful?
- What would success look like? What will their life look like in five years' time without an eating disorder, or alternatively, if the eating disorder is still sitting on their shoulders?
- If Edi is open to setting small goals, this can be helpful. Can you support them in achieving their goals? We will discuss SMART goals on page 146.

- Help them to think of all the support that is available to them and explore realistically what might make it hard to use it.
- Keep an eye out for any accommodating and/or enabling behaviours.
- What obstacles does Edi envisage up ahead? What strategies can they come up with that might address these difficulties? Help them explore and reflect on these.

"Support Edi in taking some risks. Empathize that action does not always lead to successful change."

ACTION

In this stage, individuals make actual changes to their behaviour to overcome their illness. Action involves the obvious behavioural changes and requires considerable commitment of time and energy. Strategies for this stage include:

- Offer your support in learning new strategies for coping with feelings and urges to engage in old habits or behaviours.
- Review and learn from past relapses. Make a list of signs of relapse and how Edi will address these.

- Explore how things have worked in the past.
- Assist with problem-solving.
- Support Edi in taking some risks – encourage them to set their own tasks, break goals down into manageable steps, encourage independence, encourage use of their own creative problem-solving skills, set clear limits, remind them that eating is non-negotiable and that every mistake is an opportunity for learning. Empathize that action does not always lead to successful change.
- Watch out for creeping signs of denial.
- Explore with them whether they have noticed any benefits from the small changes they have been making.
- Affirm their efforts and intentions to change.

MAINTENANCE

Maintenance is the stage in which people work to prevent or tolerate relapse. Efforts to consolidate the gains achieved during action will be made. The maintenance phase is a continuation of change. Strategies for this stage include:

- Be aware – and make a list – of signs of relapse.
- Provide support and encourage coping skills.
- Reinforce Edi's bonds with support resources. Encourage them to keep in touch with professional services, recovery groups, friends and family etc.

- Keep an eye out for signs of any creeping denial.
- Encourage new healthy interests and/or help Edi re-engage with prior healthy interests, including work, study, hobbies etc.
- Encourage more independence that can promote increased confidence.

RELAPSE

The spiral model suggests that most people who relapse do not revolve endlessly in circles and that they do not regress all the way back to where they began. Instead, each time a relapse occurs, people recycle through the stages; they potentially learn from their mistakes and can try something different the next time around. Relapse strategies include:

- Review what has been learned.
- Encourage and maintain new perspectives.
- Maintain a positive attitude.
- Regard relapse as part of the learning process.

"Each time a relapse occurs, people learn from their mistakes and can try something different the next time around."

DEFINING RECOVERY

Many carers reflect on whether Edi will ever be completely free of their eating disorder. In her *Survival Guide for Families, Friends and Sufferers*, Janet Treasure talks of the unrealistic expectations that the illness will go away after a few months whereas, in reality, after five years, approximately half the population with anorexia will have recovered, 30 per cent will remain quite severely affected by their illness, and 20 per cent will still be underweight.[25] This echoes my own experience in that it took about five years for the eating disorder to lose its grip, despite my initial insistence that I would deal with it in three months!

"Be wary of unrealistic expectations. In my own experience, it took about five years for the eating disorder to lose its grip, despite my initial insistence that I would deal with it in three months!"

People who have suffered for over five years and more, can and still do recover. Anorexia should never ever be regarded as a 'psychological tumour'. Recovery may be more challenging the

The Maudsley Model of Carer Coping

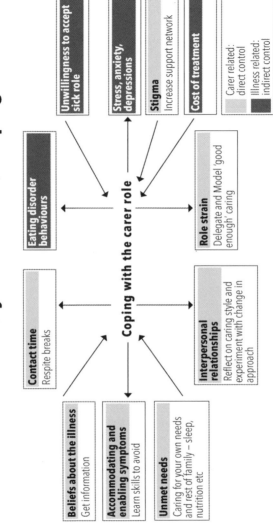

Above: The Maudsley Model of Carer Coping[27]

more entrenched it becomes, but there are cases of recovery after 20–30 years. Expectations, in terms of defining recovery, may have to be altered but it is never too late and no one should ever give up hope.

THE MAUDSLEY MODEL OF CARER COPING

Schmidt and Treasure devised The Maudsley Model of Carer Coping.[26] In it, they proposed several areas where carers can exert a greater element of control and pointed out other areas where there was less control to be had (see diagram). Whereas the darker boxes represent those areas where you, as carers, may have less control, the lighter boxes illustrate those areas where you can gain a greater sense of empowerment by applying techniques and new approaches. The New Maudsley Approach focuses their skills training techniques on those fields where you can learn new skills, such as communication techniques, the importance of looking after your own needs, encouraging reflections on where you may be accommodating or enabling the symptoms, and addressing your own beliefs about the illness and what it means for you.

COMMUNICATION STYLES

Anybody who has lived alongside somebody with an eating disorder will be only too familiar with the sheer resistance to change that accompanies the illness. In Chapter 3, we looked at the common response styles that can occur and how they can sometimes be unhelpful. So what is the best way to communicate effectively?

In the following sections we are going to look at a communication style called Motivational Interviewing (MI), a tool clinicians use in a professional setting to work *with* their patients as opposed to *against* them.

> "Two types of dialogue are 'change talk' and 'sustain talk', the latter being a person's own arguments for sustaining the status quo."

So, what is MI and how does it work? Many people are ambivalent about change. For example, they might know they should stop smoking, cut down on wine consumption, eat healthier, exercise regularly ... but choose not to. They might talk about the need to change in parallel with why it is okay to stay as they are. In MI, these two types of dialogue are known as 'change talk' and 'sustain talk', the latter being a person's own arguments for sustaining the status quo.

Here's an example of someone considering quitting smoking: *'I need to stop smoking as I want to play a better game of football, but after going out on Saturday night and smoking a pack of 20 I was up at 7 am on Sunday and played a full game.'* In this case, the individual seems to accept that quitting smoking would be a positive health move, yet follows it up immediately with sustain talk, i.e. reasons as to why it's okay to continue with his current behaviour. Most people with eating disorders respond with the 'righting reflex', in other words, nagging, cajoling, persuading, convincing ... for example, most parents will continually present a child who has an eating disorder with 1,001 reasons as to why not eating is bad for them. This is a natural response.

"Motivational Interviewing is a collaborative conversation style for strengthening a person's own motivation and commitment to change."

In reality, it is highly likely that the person will already know that their behaviour is not conducive to a healthy lifestyle, whether from external sources or their own internal voice. Consequently, when presented with another voice that takes the side of their 'change' voice, they will be more prone to balance things out by coming up with even greater 'sustain' responses. You will be met with the 'Yes … BUT … ' scenario. Furthermore, most people tend to believe themselves and trust their own opinions more than those of others. Causing someone to verbalize one side of an issue tends to move the person's balance of opinion in that direction.[28] The righting reflex, then, has the opposite effect by strengthening a person's resilience to remain with the status quo. MI is a collaborative conversation style for strengthening a person's own motivation and commitment to change.

We will explore this further in the next chapter.

6

NEW WAYS OF
COMMUNICATING

Before we begin this chapter, I would like to remind you that helping someone with an eating disorder is a steep learning curve. This chapter has an immense amount of information in it, and you are most definitely not expected to go away and become an expert in all the skills and techniques. They are there for you to dip in and dip out of, to experiment with, to change to suit your own situation, to encourage your own creativity and ability. Tuck them in your own personal toolkit. Keep a notebook; if certain techniques work, write them down and if they do not, write those down. And remember, *you are the expert.*

"You can support someone, but only they can decide whether they want to live a healthier lifestyle."

WHY MOTIVATIONAL INTERVIEWING (MI)?

Motivational Interviewing was initially developed in the field of addictions to help people who are ambivalent about change.[29] It is now used in a variety of healthcare situations, and is a skillful clinical style for eliciting from patients their own good motivations for making behaviour changes in the interest of improving their health. It involves guiding more than directing, dancing rather than wrestling, listening at least as much as telling. The overall 'spirit' has been described as collaborative (between two people), evocative (seeking out a person's own motivation and personal reserves for change), as well as recognizing and accepting the person's autonomy, i.e. they are at the helm of their own recovery process. You can support them, but only they can decide whether they want to live a healthier lifestyle.

The basic principles of MI are the use of warmth and empathy to improve a person's self-esteem along with instilling a sense of hope and confidence that change can occur. Open questions and reflective listening are used to gently challenge the ambivalence toward change. It is a useful skill to be incorporated into carer interventions. After all, you may spend a large amount of time with this person and so it is only correct that you should be trained in how best to communicate with them. Furthermore, if Edi has just had a lengthy stay in hospital, then adaptive support must continue after discharge and as a carer you should be equipped with the necessary support mechanisms.

The old Aesop's fable about the sun and the wind illustrates the superiority of persuasion over force, which is the key to MI:

The North Wind and the Sun had a quarrel about which of them was the stronger. While they were disputing with much heat and bluster, a Traveller passed along the road wrapped in a cloak. 'Let us agree,' said the Sun, 'that he is the stronger who can strip that Traveller of his cloak.'

'Very well,' growled the North Wind, and at once sent a cold, howling blast against the Traveller.

With the first gust of wind the ends of the cloak whipped about the Traveller's body. But he immediately wrapped it closely around him, and the harder the Wind blew, the tighter he held it to him. The North Wind tore angrily at the cloak, but all his efforts were in vain.

Then the Sun began to shine. At first his beams were gentle, and in the pleasant warmth after the bitter cold of the North Wind, the Traveller unfastened his cloak and let it hang loosely from his shoulders. The Sun's rays grew warmer and warmer. The man took off his cap and mopped his brow. At last he became so heated that he pulled off his cloak, and, to escape the blazing sunshine, threw himself down in the welcome shade of a tree by the roadside.

ELEMENTS OF MI

There are four interrelated elements to MI, known as PACE:

1. **P**artnership: People are their own experts. They know themselves better than anybody else. Communication, then, takes on an exploratory approach rather than an argumentative one. For example, you might say, 'So on the one hand, you talk about us starting a family – how you've always wanted to have kids of your own – yet this eating disorder is still one of the most important parts of your life. I'm curious about how the two fit in with each other.'

"Acknowledging that Edi is making an effort and has the energy to try again when things don't go according to plan helps to build and support their self-efficacy and self-esteem."

2. **A**cceptance: This does not mean you accept the behaviour. On the contrary, it means that you believe Edi has the innate capability of making the right choice for their wellbeing, allowing them to take control of their own destiny and believe that they can do it. Your belief that they can create their own goals is incredibly motivational, and with your support they can find the best path toward these goals. Carers often tell me that they find this incredibly difficult due to lack of trust and this is completely understandable. Eating disorders are deceitful and trust is an issue for all. However, acknowledging that Edi is making an effort and has the energy to try again when things don't go according to plan helps to build and support their self-efficacy and self-esteem. For example, you might say, 'You have always shown great resilience and determination throughout your life ... I have the greatest confidence in your ability to overcome this illness.'

3. **C**ompassion and empathy: People with eating disorders often feel that nobody understands them; they feel totally alone. This must be a terrifying position to be in. Try and come alongside the person that you are supporting and step into their shoes. Imagine what or how they are feeling and listen carefully to their responses. One useful exercise the New Maudsley team use during workshop training, is asking carers to fill in a form listing the activities they

engage in when they feel stressed out or uptight. The answers commonly include walking, listening to music, taking the dog out, having a few glasses of wine, talking with friends, playing bridge, shopping …. This sheet is then ripped up in front of them and they are asked to imagine somebody has just taken their coping mechanisms away. How do they feel? This is then compared with how sufferers feel when continually asked to give up their eating disorder and is a powerful exercise to promote empathy.

> "Look out for any small signs of acknowledgement that their eating disorder might be negative, notice them, repeat, and amplify this ambivalence in order to help them recognize that change might have some positive outcomes."

4. **E**vocation: Clinical psychologists Miller and Rollnick, in their book *Helping People Change,* talk about the implicit message in MI being: '*You* have what you need and together we will find it.'[30] The assumption being that people truly do have the wisdom about themselves – and the motivation and resources within themselves – to call upon. If we go back to the 'sustain talk' and 'change talk'

(see page 82), you will also recall the dangers of the 'righting reflex'. It can seem like Edi views their illness as their only true friend and ally. The harder you try to persuade or convince, the deeper they dig their heels in. However, even the most resistant person can recognize that there might be some negatives to their illness. Look out for any small signs in Edi, notice them, repeat, and amplify this ambivalence in order to help them recognize that change might have some positive outcomes. For example, you might say, 'It's interesting to hear you say that this food thing is a real pain and takes the enjoyment from planning your weekend away with your friends. I totally get that. The planning stage of a holiday is usually part of the fun.'

CORE SKILLS IN MI

The dictionary definition of 'listen' is to 'hear with attention'. In every aspect of our lives, we are required to listen. By practising and becoming aware of the key elements of active listening, we can work to build up an atmosphere of trust and respect with the person that we are listening to. Some good reasons for practitioners to hone their listening skills are listed below:

- Listening helps you to gather important information that you might otherwise miss.

- Even a little high-quality listening can greatly promote your relationship with a patient.
- Patients whose providers listen to them are more comfortable and satisfied with their care and more likely to be open and honest.
- When you take time to listen, patients feel as though you've spent a longer time with them than you actually have.
- Listening can foster change.[31]

It is interesting to reflect on how during normal communication, we tend to regularly throw a number of roadblocks in each other's way. For example, we persuade, we suggest, we question, we argue, we agree, we disagree, we interpret, we reassure, we analyse, we warn, we sympathize, we approve, we instruct, we guide, we share information ... in fact, sometimes, it seems we do everything *but* truly listen!

One of the core basic skills in MI is the acronym known as 'OARS', which stands for:

- **O**pen questions
- **A**ffirmations
- **R**eflections
- **S**ummaries

Try to keep this acronym in mind during communication.

OPEN QUESTIONS

Asking open rather than closed questions invites the person to expand on their response as opposed to giving short 'Yes' or 'No' answers. For example:

- 'How can I be the best support to you in your recovery path?'
- 'What would help you?'

Note that MI trainers always recommend never asking more than three questions in a row.

AFFIRMATIONS

These are a way of praising, recognizing the person's strengths, efforts, and abilities. For example:

- 'That must have been difficult for you … Thanks for sharing that with me.'
- 'You've done a really good job of dealing with your anxiety tonight.'
- 'You've tried really hard this week.'

The New Maudsley team recommends praising the process, not the outcome. Recognizing the person's effort – the challenges they encounter, for example – is more motivational than the end result. Affirmations beginning with 'I' should also be avoided as these tend to focus more on the person providing the affirmation. 'I'm really proud of you,' for example, can sound a bit patronizing or be interpreted as having parental overtones and result in resistance. You can even use affirmations for a joint discussion with Edi, i.e., discuss each other's strengths, past success, and efforts in particular projects.

"Reflective listening is a way of showing the person that you are *really* listening to them."

REFLECTIONS

Reflective listening provides proof of 'active listening' and helps deepen understanding by clarifying any misunderstandings. For example:

- 'It sounds as if what you're saying is that you feel that you don't deserve to ...'
- 'You feel that going out to eat on your birthday will really increase your anxiety ...'
- 'You're very frightened of going back to school because ...'

It has been said that real, authentic listening is the best gift somebody can give another person, but unfortunately it does not come naturally to most of us. When someone is telling us something, we are often thinking of how to respond. Perhaps we have an example of our own we want to share, or know of someone else who has gone through a similar experience. Reflective listening is a way of showing the person that you are *really* listening to them.

SUMMARIES

A summary is a collection of reflections and can be used to pull together responses to check whether you understand what you have heard. They also provide the opportunity for the recipient to add anything that the listener may have missed. For example:

'So just let me pull that together to make sure I'm understanding you. You've been really gearing up for going out for your birthday tonight. You called the restaurant a couple of days ago to check on the menu and you chose options that you think you'll feel comfortable with. However, you're now beginning to feel quite anxious about the evening. You say that you'd be really disappointed in yourself if you didn't go and you're getting a bit panicky as to whether you'll be able to handle it once you get there, especially with your mum and dad also being there. The last thing you want is to cause a scene, especially as your mum gets a bit uptight over the whole thing. Anything else that I've missed?'

Summaries are a recap of what the person has just said. They also give the recipient the opportunity to fill in any gaps you may have missed or correct any misinterpretations. I remember going to a motivational interviewing conference a few years ago where the clinical psychologist Bill Miller gave a wonderful description of a summary by asking us to imagine a field or a meadow of wildflowers and weeds. In a summary we pick out those reflections that may possibly elicit change thoughts; in other words, we distinguish the wildflowers from the weeds and hand back the posy of wildflowers.

Let's now look at some of those core skills in a bit more detail, beginning with the fundamental MI skill of listening.

LISTENING

Reflections can either be simple or complex. A simple reflection generally repeats back to the person what the listener has heard without adding any additional meaning or interpretation.

Complex reflections, on the other hand, tend to add more strength, i.e., they include the listener's own interpretation of what they have heard. This can elicit different responses. The speaker may disagree entirely with the listener's interpretation or alternatively, it may encourage the speaker to pause for thought … In other words, this new interpretation may sow a new seed. The listener may be better able to hear what they themselves are thinking and then continue to elaborate. Clinical psychologists, Miller and Rollnick recommend thinking of simple and complex reflections like an iceberg. A simple reflection is limited to what shows above the water, the content that has already been expressed, whereas a complex reflection makes a guess about what lies beneath the surface.[32]

Here are some examples of simple and complex reflections when the opportunity to use them arises:

Edi: *I just feel so alone in all of this, like there's no future … no way out.*

Mum: *You feel there's no way out right now.*

(**Simple reflection involves repeating back, not adding much to utterance.**)

OR

Mum: *You feel trapped and lonely, with nobody to turn to and you can't see any light at the end of the tunnel.*

(**Complex reflection involves adding more strength, i.e. Mum's interpretation of utterance.**)

Edi: *I don't deserve to eat dinner tonight. I only ran a couple of miles and I usually run five.*

Partner: *So because you didn't run as far as you usually run, you don't deserve to eat.*

(**Simple reflection involves repeating back, not adding much to utterance.**)

OR

Partner: *That anorexic* voice is really bullying you tonight. It acts as a real tyrant to your wellbeing.
   (Complex reflection involves adding more strength.)

> "You will come to recognize when opportunities arise. I always referred to them as 'golden opportunities'."

Remember, your entire pattern of communication should not be focused on using simple and complex reflections, or MI in general. This is both unsustainable and unrealistic. Even professional therapists only work with their clients for the best part of an hour. You will come to recognize when opportunities arise. I always referred to them as 'golden opportunities', i.e., when my daughter opened up and wanted to talk about her feelings, her illness, her future …

QUESTIONING

It will probably be no surprise to you that closed questions that elicit monosyllabic answers should be avoided in favour of open questions that promote the opportunity for Edi to speak and elaborate on how they are feeling. Overall, as suggested earlier, questions should be limited (never more than three in a row), otherwise it may feel like an interrogation exercise. When using MI in a professional setting, therapists aim for a ratio of 2:1 reflections:questions. Remember, voice tone is also important when working with open questions. Questions, for example, should be asked in a non-judgemental manner with no sarcastic undertones.

Here are some examples of open and closed questions:

Edi: *I just feel so alone in all of this, like there's no future …
no way out.*

Sister: *Do you feel lonely all of the time?*

(**Closed question eliciting a yes/no answer**)

OR

Sister: *That must really suck. How can I help you feel less
isolated?*

(**Open question eliciting greater elaboration**)

Edi: *You make me feel different from the others in our family.*

Dad: *I guess your illness makes me more protective. Does
that make you uncomfortable?*

(**Closed question eliciting a yes/no answer**)

OR

Dad: *That's interesting you say that. In what ways do I make
you feel different?*

(**Open question eliciting greater elaboration**)

CASE STUDY

The following short scenario illustrates OARS being used in practice.

Jess is leaving home in the next few weeks to go to college where she will share an apartment with three friends. Her parents, Paula and David, have been working toward achieving a more collaborative approach and now feel more confident working with Jess and supporting her recovery. They want to sit down and discuss Jess's plans for how she will cope with meal plans once she is no longer living at home full-time.

Paula: Jess, do you mind if we sit down for 20 minutes or so and talk about your meal plans once you head off in a couple of weeks? (**Closed question**)

Jess: Not really a great time, Mum.

David: There's never going to be a perfect time, honey. Mum and I understand that this sort of talk makes you feel uncomfortable. (**Complex reflection**) *We've watched you work so hard over the last few months to improve your health and this next move is a really positive new chapter in your life that you thoroughly deserve. It's going to be an exciting time ahead for you.* (**Affirmation**) *I know you must feel some sort of nervousness around the food issue and mum and I would like to support you, perhaps listen to your plans and see how we can help in some way. How do* *you feel about switching off your laptop and having a chat about that?* (**Open question**)

Jess: *(sigh) There's not really much to discuss. I'm more than capable of sticking with the meal plan. You've watched me work with it for months.*

Paula: *We're picking up on a bit of frustration; you don't really want to be focusing on your eating disorder when there are more exciting plans up ahead. You've done brilliantly, Jess. There have been challenges along the way – you've really braved the storm and got on with it.* (**Affirmation**) *Having been with you from the very start, Dad and I too have some concerns as to the next phase. We're really excited for you and you've worked damned hard to get to this point. On the other hand, we've always been here to support you through the tougher times, and it would be really helpful for us to hear what your thoughts are with regards to how you might deal with any potential difficulties and where you can access helpful support if you should need it. We trust that you are more than capable of addressing any hurdles and you know you can always rely on us to support you in any way we can.*

(Mum uses complex reflections, praise, and affirmations. She's also honest and open in admitting to concerns that they may have. She reminds Jess of the collaborative nature of recovery and how they are always there to support her.)

Jess: *I'm not the first person with an eating disorder to go off to college, you know! I'll manage fine.*

David: Fair enough ... It sounds like you have no concerns at all then. (**Complex reflection**)

Jess: Well I'd be lying if I said I didn't have SOME concerns. Obviously, there are SOME!

David: Yeah, that's understandable – living away from home for the first time is a big step for all people your age. Recovering from an eating disorder may add an extra challenging layer. What do you think? (**Complex reflection + open question**)

Jess: Well, apart from going away in the first place, I'm a bit concerned about how we'll manage food, whether we'll share the cooking ... I want to buy my own food and cook on my own but I also want to be part of the new experience. No point in hiding myself away, I should be staying at home if that's the case ...

Paula: So you're feeling a bit apprehensive about how you're going to keep to your meal plan and how you'll fit your needs around their routines. (**Complex reflection**)

Jess: Yeah, kind of ... I mean breakfast will be okay, we'll all have different schedules and be going out at different times, so we'll fix things ourselves. Lunch should be the same. To be honest it's just dinner that I'm a bit nervous about. Chloe has already said how much she's looking forward to cooking and eating together in the evening.

David: And that's worrying you a bit. (**Complex reflection**) I have some suggestions but I'm sure you're giving it good thought on your own as to solutions. (**Affirmation and**

recognizing autonomy) *What sort of eating set-up would make you feel less anxious?* (**Open question**)

Jess: Well, I don't like junk food … anything fatty or creamy or too oily … and I still find eating meat a bit difficult and I don't think that's going to change between then and now.

Paula: Okay, so you're frightened that you're not all going to have the same tastes – that there are some foods that some people will like and others won't. (**Complex reflection**)

Jess: I know that one of the other girls doesn't eat red meat. She eats chicken and fish though.

Paula: You've said before that your roommates also know about your eating difficulties. (**Simple reflection**)

Jess: Yeah, they do and Chloe has been a really great friend so I'm sure she'll understand if there are some hiccups. I'm also planning on coming home on weekends, especially in the first few weeks.

Paula: So that's another option. I could also drive down with some food – casseroles, and so forth. (**Accommodating and enabling behaviour**)

Jess: Muuuummmm!

Paula: Sorry, you're right. Thanks for flagging up my kangaroo tendencies! Anyway, we're right behind you and we'll look forward to seeing you on weekends. Well done for thinking ahead. (**Affirmation + reaffirming collaborative support**)

SUMMARY OF MI

An inadherent MI style includes:
- Arguing, disagreeing, or challenging
- Judging, criticizing, blaming, sarcasm
- Warning of negative consequences
- Using logic
- Using defensiveness
- Advice that is not asked for or advice that is likely to fall on deaf ears
- Asserting authority
- Direct confrontation

Meanwhile, an adherent MI approach involves:
- Asking whether Edi would like some advice. For example, 'I read an interesting article yesterday by a guy who'd recently recovered from anorexia. Can I share some of the things he talked about?'
- Affirming or praising. For example, 'You've always shown such determination and stamina. You've really fought back with all of your characteristic strength and determination.'
- Emphasizing a person's autonomy. For example, 'Only you can do this. I can support you but you're at the helm in terms of your recovery.'
- Using empathy. For example, 'You've a lot going on in your life right now. It can't be easy with all your exams coming up and fighting an eating disorder at the same time.'

RECOGNIZING CHANGE TALK

Let's now look again at recognizing change talk and sustain talk (see page 82). Ambivalence about change is a regular theme when working with someone with an eating disorder. Any talk that may hint at change can be very quickly swapped with talk that retains the status quo.[33] You may hear regular intentions to change, such as, 'I must stick with my meal plan this week.' However, such statements do not necessarily mean that this will happen. The key question, then, is how can *you* encourage or elicit change talk?

REMEMBER

Do not get too tied up with identifying every utterance that comes out of Edi's mouth. It is more about being able to recognize potential change talk when it does come. For me, the slightest hint of a golden opportunity resulted in everything being dropped and the listening ear being switched on at full volume!

DARN-CATS:

The elements of change talk can be explained using the acronym, DARN-CATS:

Desire to want to change. For example, 'I do want to feel better and get my life back.'

Ability – the person's self-perceived ability about whether they can achieve the desired behaviour. For example, 'I'd like to go out to dinner with the family this weekend but I'm not sure I can do it.'

Reasons to change – when the person comes up with reasons as to why change *might* be helpful. For example, 'I might feel less tired and cold; I might be able to join my friends on holiday when school breaks up.' Notice that this type of talk implies neither desire nor ability.

Need to change – this represents urgency or importance for behaviour change. For example, 'I need to … ', 'I must …', 'I can't keep on like this …'.

Whilst preparatory change talk reflects the pro-side of ambivalence, mobilizing change talk moves more toward actions in favour of change, in other words, **C**ommitment.

Commitment talk signals the likelihood of action taking place in the near future. For example, 'I want to call my doctor in the morning and ask for an appointment to talk about this. I seriously need to consider going back into hospital to fight this thing.'

Activation talk is when the person suggests that they are moving toward action. For example, 'I am ready to go back into hospital; I am prepared to do whatever it takes this time to recover once and for all.'

Taking **S**teps indicates that the first signs of action have been completed. For example, 'I called my doctor yesterday and I have an appointment with the eating disorder team next week; I've asked my husband to sit with me every mealtime and we've already come up with a list of distractions that may help me feel less anxious.'

EVOKING PREPARATORY CHANGE TALK

The key question, then, that all carers will want to ask is how they can help promote change talk or build motivation in Edi so that they might want to think about change. There is usually more commitment to change if the person is talking about this themselves as opposed to other people doing it for them, so asking open questions is a step in the right direction.

ACTIVITY:
Looking at Options

DARN-CATS can be a useful tool to open conversations and to help both carers and Edi visualize and verbalize options. Below are some examples of questions you might ask:

Desire

- 'What sort of life do you hope for in, say, five years' time?'
- 'What are you looking for from your therapy?'

- What do you hope will happen after you've completed your therapy?

Ability

- 'What changes do you think you could handle this week?'
- 'What would be manageable?'
- 'How confident are you that you can put these in place?'

Reasons

- 'What reasons can you see for running fewer kilometres/miles every day?'
- 'What might be some of the good things about easing up on the pressures you place on yourself?'

Need

- 'How important is it for you to follow your meal plan?'
- 'What do you need to do?'
- 'What support do you need to help you through this?'

Any aspect of DARN can be used on a readiness ruler (see page 109) to check out discrepancies between thinking and acting, or ambivalence regarding change. Questions such as these can activate the person toward change, eliciting his or her own motivations to change and fostering their own creative ideas on how they can make this happen.

ACTIVITY:
Using the Readiness Ruler

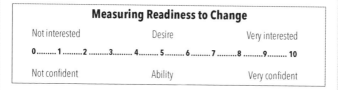

Measuring Readiness to Change		
Not interested	Desire	Very interested
0.........1.........2.........3.........4.........5.........6.........7.........8.........9.........10		
Not confident	Ability	Very confident

Consider the following questions in the context of your *own* need to experiment with change in terms of your own approach to the eating disorder:

- How ready are you to leave your position in 'Action' to come alongside Edi at whatever stage they are at, so you can work with them for change?
- Where do you think Edi would mark themselves in terms of importance and confidence to make changes?
- Use the ruler and DARN to begin a conversation with another carer within your family, or with Edi.

REMEMBER

Coming alongside Edi is not the same as agreeing with them and their eating disorder behaviours. It is getting them to reflect on where they are and sowing the seed that change might be an option in the future. Contemplating change is a big step for all of us. The readiness ruler and DARN-CATS can be useful tools to accompany OARS (see page 92) to open conversations and to help to visualize and verbalize options. The more an individual can visualize and verbalize something, the more likely it is to happen.

ACTIVITY:
The Decisional Balance

When faced with ambivalence, a useful exercise is the decisional balance, which is a 2 x 2 matrix that lists the pros and cons of change. It can help to explore ambivalence and be used to reflect on how to go about generating change thoughts or talk. If Edi is willing, this can be an effective way of reflecting and, hopefully, encouraging change talk.

Pros of No Change	Cons of No Change
E.g. My eating disorder keeps me safe and in control.	E.g. It stops me enjoying life … my friends, my family, social life.
Pros of Change	Cons of Change
E.g. I would feel healthier, less cold, more energy. I'd get my life back again.	E.g. I would feel really, really frightened. I may never stop eating.

For further discussion on the use of the decisional balance tool, take a look at this link on YouTube: https://www.youtube.com/watch?v=7vJ8jBqzVqU

DEVELOPING DISCREPANCY

This can be a useful tool in communicating with Edi to highlight any discrepancies between current behaviour and values, and future plans, goals etc. It can encourage Edi to reflect on any differences between where they are today and where they want to be in the future.

Edi's current behaviour is likely to hold them back and reduce the likelihood that they can achieve whatever life goals they envisage for themselves. You can help to motivate them to resolve the discrepancy through behavioural change.

CASE STUDY

Cheryl wants to go ahead with a holiday to Australia with her best friend Anya. There are some concerns for Anya: how is it going to happen if Cheryl is too weak, if she's too rigid around food, if she's really unhappy and filled with anxiety with anything that is out of the ordinary? Anya helps Cheryl explore these discrepancies:

Cheryl: I am so looking forward to our trip to Australia next year. I just feel I'm dealing with so much at the moment. I feel like getting away right now. I wish I'd saved up enough so we could go this year.

Anya: I'm really looking forward to our trip too. We've spoken about it long enough, not to mention saved up for it! You've put a fantastic travel plan together. **(Affirmation)** *I'm also really excited about it. I feel we can have so much. fun on this trip, yet I have a few concerns over your health. I really admire how you're dealing with your challenges, you know, like seeking out professional help. The eating behaviours still seem as if they're a bit of a challenge for you; you've mentioned that yourself. It would be useful to know how I could be a better support to you in the months ahead. What do you think?* **(Developing discrepancy between future goals and current behaviour/Praise/ Affirmation/Ending with open question)**

Of course, Edi may be aware of the discrepancy between their current behaviour and any future plans or goals. If it was so easy, then why don't they see the need to change and act on that need? There may be several reasons:

1. The discrepancy may be too large and daunting, which is why they recommend taking small steps.
2. They may not have the confidence to think change is possible and feel that there's no way they can possibly change.
3. The thought of change can be so painful that Edi uses denial or avoidance simply as a self-defense mechanism. This will be exacerbated particularly if accompanied by 1) and 2).

Obviously, making Edi feel miserable about themself is always going to be counter-productive to recovery. Supporting them to consider discrepancy without the pain will require empathic, non-judgemental communication, whilst taking into account the four interrelated aspects of MI (see page 88). Be curious and creative – experiment with using discrepancy. Look at what works and what doesn't work. Allow what doesn't work to inform any future approaches.

7

ADVANCING YOUR COMMUNICATION SKILLS

Once you feel comfortable using what you learned in the previous chapter, you can experiment with more advanced MI and questioning techniques. The techniques are challenging, but you might find that you are a naturally empathic listener. In my early years as a researcher, we trained 'expert carers', i.e., those people with first-hand experience of supporting someone with an eating disorder, to coach other carers. Although the professionals attained higher levels of proficiency in MI, we found that the expert carers still reached basic proficiency levels.[34]

REMEMBER

If it takes you time to get the hang of these techniques, don't be hard on yourself. Remember, we learn from mistakes. If a particular response did not work for you, reflect on it, learn from it. How could you work with the same scenario if it occurs again?

Carers often comment that communicating in this way, with a new awareness and using the techniques, feels abnormal or strange. However, remember living with anorexia is not a normal situation. Each family, couple, relationship has their own particular conversational dynamics. Try and work these techniques in with your own form of dialogue.

ADVANCED LISTENING TECHNIQUES

DOUBLE-SIDED REFLECTION

Reflecting ambivalence is used for developing discrepancy in the sufferer's values and future goals. For example, 'On the one hand … yet on the other hand …' Edi may recognize the need to change, but be at a loss as to how they can instigate change. Here's an example:

Sister: *You said last week that you wanted to think of new ways of trying to talk with Mum and Dad that didn't end in carnage. How's that been going?* (**Simple reflection/Open question**)

Edi: *Not very well, really. I was trying to talk more openly about all this stuff … I think I've been struggling a bit as well … It's not easy. Talking about university, for example, it started off well, but then they were trying yet again to give me advice and I just started screaming at them, 'My whole life is always going to be a mess', and Mum starts crying, so same old, same old …*

Sister: *So, on one level, you're prepared to open up these subjects and discuss possible plans for the future, yet on another level you find it really difficult when Mum and Dad say the wrong thing or you feel perhaps you're being pushed too quickly.* (**Reflection using developing discrepancy**)

SHIFTING FOCUS

Sometimes you may have to change the subject to keep Edi on track. Here's an example:

Edi: *I just feel so frustrated – Mum and Dad want to know EVERYTHING about my life – what I eat, where I'm going when I go out, when I'll be home, where I exercise, how much I exercise … It really feels like I have no choices. I have no other place to live. All they seem to concentrate on is food and every morsel that goes into my mouth.*

Sister: *I can feel your frustration, I really can. It sounds really upsetting for you. You probably think you have the hard end of the stick compared to me when it comes to intrusion right now. I'm not surprised you feel angry and frustrated. You're probably feeling pretty sad as well because it didn't used to be like this for you. I'm not sure how to tackle that one. Do you mind if we come back to that later and for now let's just chat about something else? How do you feel about having a little chat about the choices you feel that you do have?* (**Affirmation/ Empathy/Complex reflection/Shifting focus/Open question**)

CITING WITH THE NEGATIVE

This involves taking the negative side of the argument, or even amplifying it. Here's an example:

Edi: I hate these winter mornings … It's harder running against the cold wind.

Husband: Your daily exercise routine sounds a bit of a grind to you. What would happen if you thought about skipping it on days like this when the weather is bad? (**Complex reflection/ Open question**)

Edi: I don't know. Guilty, I guess … guilty and bad about myself, lazy … no self-control.

Husband: Hmm … that's too bad. So skipping it isn't an option right now. Giving it a miss for today would cause you too much anxiety; it would be too much for you to tolerate. (**Empathy/Reflection/Citing with the negative**)

Edi: Mmm … I guess … it freaks me out when I don't exercise. It does help the anxiety, but it's just so cold and miserable out there. I don't know how much longer I can push myself like this. (**Edi may still go out, despite her husband's response. However, by responding in a more non-confrontational manner, he may have encouraged her to consider more self-compassion to address her anxiety.**)

When citing with the negative, be careful not to use sarcasm or be aggressive. If there's sarcasm or aggression, it can have the opposite effect.

REFRAMING

This is when you encourage Edi to see something in a different way, taking something they are unhappy with and reframing it in a more positive light. Here's an example:

Mum: *Self-control is important to you, but at the same time it also weighs heavily on your shoulders, making you do things that you don't particularly feel like doing.* (**Complex reflection using developing discrepancy**)

Edi: *Sometimes it feels that way.*

Mum: *This part of your personality has been positive in many areas of your life – you play the piano beautifully and you certainly needed to be disciplined to have achieved this. Your music also alleviates some of your anxiety.* (**Affirmation/ Complex reflection**)

Edi: *That' s true.*

Mum: *On the one hand self-control can be your friend, but it can also act as your enemy.* (**Complex reflection using reframing**)

AGREEMENT WITH A TWIST

This is a reflection or an acknowledgement, followed by reframing. Here's an example:

Partner: *Dinner is less stressful if you can find exactly the right ingredients and safe foods that don't freak you out. However, this usually means having to go to quite a few* different supermarkets on your way back from work. It must be worth the effort though? (**Complex reflection + Reframe**)

Edi: On some levels, yes, but a lot of the time, no … Some days I feel tired and quite pissed off that I have to go through all this rigmarole when other normal people don't. Most nights it doesn't even work.

EMPHASIZING PERSONAL CHOICE

Making choices for other people rarely works. It is more likely to encourage resistance and deceit as well as stirring up resentment. I am sure we have all come across people who just love to tell us what to do. It may be our parents, certain friends, colleagues, or our boss. Advice and guidance are useful, but there are ways to offer them without it sounding as if we know better. For someone with an eating disorder whose self-esteem is low anyway, it can often send a subtle message that they are not quite up to it when it comes to finding their own way. Of course, you probably feel that this is indeed the case – the trick is to avoid kangaroo responses (see page 58) by nudging Edi to come up with their own solutions.

Mum: I realize that you are in charge of your own recovery and that I can merely support you in your fight. You have choices – you talk of your longing to be like your other friends. You've also spoken about your desire never to have to go back into the in-patient unit again. You sound understandably *frightened and distressed at the anorexia taking a stronger and stronger hold of you. What steps can you take to feel a bit more empowered?* (**Summary/Open question, emphasizing personal choice**)

Edi: *I'm not sure. I'm starting to feel a bit overwhelmed, to be honest.*

Mum: *You've worked so hard to get this point. I can imagine it's a pretty confusing and frightening time for you.* (**Affirmation/Empathy**)

ADVANCED QUESTIONING TECHNIQUES

The following advanced questioning techniques are part of the advanced training course for the MI practitioner. You may find some of these questioning techniques useful. The most important point for you to remember is that these techniques can take years for professionals to master. The point here is to play around and experiment with them.

LEADING QUESTIONS

It can sometimes be tempting to ask leading questions that have the desired answer already embedded in them. Questions such as, 'Don't you think that … ?', 'Have you thought about … ?' or 'What about trying … ?' lead Edi to believe that you have all the best answers, as discussed above, and they will therefore be less likely to come up with their own solutions or to accept ownership of the decision that has been made.

Furthermore, it may come across as if it is your agenda that dominates, with Edi being cast in the role of passive recipient, a situation likely to result in a wall of resistance, as well as being frustrating for you. Asking permission beforehand is motivationally adherent, such as asking if they can make a suggestion, especially if they appear to be stuck. For example, 'This may or may not work but what do you think about this idea …?'

'WHY' QUESTIONS

Use 'why' questions very carefully as they can evoke a defensive response that comes across as critical and disapproving. For example, questions such as, 'Why did you respond in this way?' may suggest to Edi that they need to justify themselves, which again can result in greater resistance or ambivalence. A more effective way would be to use a reflection, followed by an open question: 'I found what you said about … interesting. Tell me more about that.'

QUESTIONS THAT CLARIFY

These questions are useful when there is uncertainty as to what Edi means. They also offer the opportunity to clarify any misunderstandings or misinterpretations. Here's an example:

Let me know if I'm hearing you right. You say you're becoming more and more frightened at your increasing need to exercise more and how you're starting to feel really panicky right after work due to a strong need to go to straight to the gym. Is that a fair recap?

QUESTIONS THAT CHALLENGE LIMITING BELIEFS

Comments from people suffering from an eating disorder frequently reflect limiting beliefs. For example, they might say, 'I could never do that', 'I'll never get better, I'm just not sure I have the confidence to make it happen', 'I'm at a loss as to what to do next'.

Negative beliefs that people hold about themselves or their situation prevent them from moving forward. Careful questioning techniques can challenge and highlight limiting beliefs. By combining reflections and affirmations with motivationally adherent and empathic responses, you can skillfully weave open questions into the dialogue before becoming more focused on, and specific about, the belief that is preventing Edi from moving forward.

A useful technique to challenge limiting beliefs is to encourage the person to suspend this thought for a while, i.e., to become more creative in coming up with a possible solution. Here are some examples:

- 'How would you advise a friend who had the same problem?
- 'What beliefs would you need to adopt in order for this to happen?'

REFRAMING NEGATIVES TO POSITIVES

Intertwined with limiting beliefs, there may be a display of low self-esteem. Individuals may, for example, become critical of themselves and/or of others. This not only occurs with people who suffer from an eating disorder, but also with those who are supporting them. In this short dialogue, it is the carer who needs some support. Joe has noticed increasing negative self-talk from a friend who is supporting his wife through her eating disorder. He tries to motivate him to get back on track by reframing negatives to positives.

Carer: I mean every day it's apparent that there's something that I'm not doing right, something that I've said that comes out wrong. I do go away and analyse what's happened, especially after she has a meltdown and I feel I'm to blame.

Joe: From what you've been saying, you're doing a stellar job of coming up with new strategies, walking away from those meltdowns etc. It can't be an easy situation! You also sound as if you're learning a lot from the times when things perhaps don't go so well and using that to inform the next time.

Carer: *I've made a bucketful of mistakes, but I suppose I am learning … slowly.*

Joe: *You've got some stamina. I'm sure lots of people would have thrown in the towel by now. You're living in challenging circumstances every day, yet you've found time to research eating disorders, joined support groups and you mentioned using the skills from your support groups has made an impact on your relationship with Anna. Well done to both of you – you make a great team.*

CHALLENGING QUESTIONS

Individuals suffering from an eating disorder frequently become negative and use destructive language. Through a series of affirmations, reflections, and questions, MI techniques can challenge these negative generalizations and perceptions in a given situation. In this next brief dialogue, Edi is questioning her dad's attitude to her. Dad gives lots of praise and uses open questions to explore the source of the emotions. He does not talk about his own emotions and needs, but instead provides a firm accepting stance for his daughter to say things that could be unhelpfully construed as personally attacking and hurtful.

Edi: *You make me feel very depressed. I feel that I'm an absolutely crap person. Why do you still insist on helping me? I'm just not worth it. You'd be better off without me.*

Dad: *I'm sorry that you feel that way. It certainly isn't our intention to make you feel like that. You're a very special young woman, not only to your family, but to so many other people. I'm interested in hearing what makes you feel this way.*

Edi: *I just feel responsible for all that I put you through. I do try to follow meal plans and act 'normally', but it always seems to go pear-shaped at the littlest thing ... I just feel like a hopeless loser, bringing angst to everything and everybody.*

Dad: *You're working really hard fighting back against this monster that's continually screaming in your ear. It must be really difficult for you and we're proud of the way you're fighting against it and working with your team. We're all here for you all the way, as you would be for any of us. We're going to be*

REMEMBER

The skills and techniques within the New Maudsley Approach represent a steep learning curve. Dip in and dip out of them. You are not going to get it right all the time. None of us do ... whether in the New Maudsley Approach or any other part of life, come to think of it! Learn from mistakes, experiment with them and, above all, be kind to yourself. Supporting someone with an eating disorder is not easy. Change is difficult for Edi and changing your responses is also challenging.

standing right alongside you in your battle against it and we will come out the other side with you. I get the feeling that the more you head toward your target weight, the louder this monster screams at you.

Edi: *I feel it's forcing me to face up to how I feel, and I've not done that for a while. My survival strategy is that I just don't think about that sort of stuff.*

MI IN PRACTICE

On page 88, we looked at the four interrelated aspects of MI spirit known as PACE: partnership, acceptance, compassion, evocation. The following sub-sections use PACE as a backdrop for addressing common scenarios that carers frequently find themselves up against when supporting someone with an eating disorder.

> "Accept their autonomy – they are at the helm of their own recovery path and trust that they will get there."

SUPPORTING SELF-EFFICACY

As we said earlier, people are their own experts and it is important for you, as a carer, to bear this in mind in your communication with Edi. Consequently, when trying to elicit change talk, it is important how we go about doing it. I'm sure you'll agree that advice, lectures, and even gentle guidance can often be met with a great big wall of resistance and a hundred and one questions as to why you've got the wrong end of the stick, that there's nothing wrong or that you're exaggerating, that you don't know anything about their situation or how they are feeling. Promoting self-efficacy, on the other hand, refers to your belief in Edi that they can and will have the ability to carry out and succeed with a specific task. In other words, to accept their autonomy, i.e. that they are at the helm of their own recovery path and that you trust that they will get there. Here's an example:

Brother: Last night you said that when Mum insisted that you clear your plate you felt overwhelming anxiety. (**Simple reflection**)

Edi: Yeah, I just can't handle it. That way of dealing with the situation just does not help me at all.

Brother: Yeah, it must be exhausting for you having this turmoil night after night. I can sense it when talking to you. You're pretty smart too though and I know and trust that you'll be only too aware that everybody needs to eat to live. What do you think the options are? (**Open question**)

Edi: All I need is for you all to be quiet; don't say anything because everybody nagging on at me just makes it worse and then I get so friggin' angry.

Brother: *It sounds like a really shitty situation for you. You sound frightened and angry.* (**Complex reflection – people with eating disorders have difficulties accepting and managing emotions and so reflections that can bring emotions to the forefront are particularly helpful**)

Edi: *… and then when Mum started her nagging last night, ah geez … I felt myself growing more and more annoyed and I really needed to try so hard to calm myself down. If I hadn't managed to do that, she could have ended up wearing the casserole sauce, I swear!*

Brother: *That wouldn't have gone down well – they've just painted the kitchen (laugh). Good for you though, that you managed to calm yourself down. You didn't used to be able to do that as well.* (**Rolling with resistance using humour**) *Still not much fun for you. I'm just wondering whether you can think of anything that can be done as a distraction to make dinnertimes less frightening? You always come up with great ideas for everybody else's difficulties!* (**Supporting self-efficacy using empathy/Emphasizing personal choice/Open question/ Affirmation**)

EXPRESSING EMPATHY

By using empathy, combined with reflective listening, your aim is to understand Edi's feelings and perspectives without judgement, criticism, or blame. You are not sympathizing with them, nor are you agreeing with them. You are trying to accept their challenges and understand what it must be like living in their shoes.

Edi: *All you want me to do is to eat and you just can't understand that I am healthy, I do not want to eat HUGE dinners and that I'm happy with my life as it is!*

Mum: *It's hard on you. I can see that.* (**Empathy**) *I know you hate falling out with us, and it must feel as if it's a constant battle with this other voice telling you to act in a different manner.* (**Developing discrepancy**) *It must take a lot of strength to fight your frustration and fear.* (**Empathy plus acknowledging and praising the efforts**)

DISCORD

Edi may be extremely resistant to change and become extremely upset, especially if they feel they are being pushed into a corner. Lecturing, arguing, pestering, and nagging can quickly result in huge arguments and distress for all concerned. I'm sure you can relate to that feeling of living on a knife edge or walking on eggshells. It is tremendously exhausting for all concerned. When emotions are running high, it can be useful to notice this and take a step back. This does not mean you intend to ignore the behaviour or issues you were discussing. However, it will be more beneficial coming back to talk about it later when the emotional climate is calmer. Think of a wave – you don't want to address the issue when the wave is picking up speed, nor do you want to continue at the crest of the wave. Wait until the wave has broken and the water is calm once again.

Clinical psychologists, Miller and Rollnick, use the term 'discord' to encapsulate resistance and list its many guises:

- **Defending** themself by blaming someone else – 'It's your fault, you cause this drama every mealtime by insisting I eat this crap', by minimizing – 'I'm not the sick anorexic you all make me out to be, I'm pretty healthy', by justifying their behaviour – 'Why are you guys nagging me? I'm trying to live healthily. If I catch COVID, I'll have a much better chance of not having to be hospitalized if I'm not fat. Read the news!'
- **Challenging stance** or taking an opposite stance – 'You really have no idea about where I'm coming from, do you?', 'You're wrong and I'm right!', 'You say you are here to support me. Well … I don't need support like this.'
- **Talking over you or interrupting –** 'I've heard enough', 'Sorry, I don't care how much you rant on, I'm doing it my way.'
- **Disengaging** when the fog comes over. You are talking and it is obvious that Edi is somewhere else. They may act distracted or their eyes may glaze over. Whatever occurs, they have obviously shut off.[35]

When there is discord, particularly when it is accompanied by high emotion, it is often better to take time out – to walk away, if it is safe to do so. Here's an example of what you might say:

Partner: *You are extremely upset right now. We're not getting anywhere when we're arguing like this. You're emotional, I'm emotional, the kids are upstairs listening to all this. We are not going to arrive at any solution whilst we're in this state of mind. I'm going to go out for a short walk just to clear my head. Let's talk about this later when we both feel a bit better. I love you very much. I hope you know that. Your safety and wellbeing is so important to us all.* **(Rolling with resistance by using reflections and affirmations)**

"Affirmations help to reduce tension and defensiveness."

There are several ways of dealing with discord. Apologizing, affirming, and shifting focus are examples. Saying 'sorry', if you feel you are to blame, emphasizes the collaborative nature of the relationship and sends the message that you are not perfect, it is natural to get things wrong at times, and the world still spins. Affirmations, on the other hand, help to reduce tension and defensiveness. Shifting focus involves either taking some temporary time-out or changing the subject, if appropriate.

GIVING INFORMATION AND ASKING PERMISSION

As discussed above, advice and guidance feel like the most natural way in the world when caring for somebody with an eating disorder. 'Why can't you just eat?', 'Why are you doing this to yourself?', 'I have a fact list about anorexia here and I'd like you to read it', 'The brain needs so many calories alone to function. You really need to eat a bit more.' Unfortunately, as many of you will know only too well, advice-giving tends to fall on deaf ears or result in a wall of resistance being thrown up. In MI, there are ways in which therapists work with advice giving.

Asking permission

Giving information is totally fine if Edi asks for it or is open to receiving it. However, as already stated, it is most likely to elicit resistance if they are not ready or unwilling to receive it. In general, it is fine to inform when Edi asks you to do so, but giving solutions or advice should be avoided.

A second way is to ask permission, e.g., 'I read an interesting report on eating disorders in a magazine. Would you like to hear what it said?', 'May I make a suggestion?', 'Would it be all right for me to tell you one concern I have about this plan?'

There may be information or advice that you feel ethically obliged to give Edi. You can still use autonomy and supportive language that acknowledges Edi's right to agree or disagree with your information. For example, 'I don't know whether this applies to you, but ...', 'You may agree or disagree with what I'm about to say ...', You may or may not find this article information useful ...'.

> "Generally, the more directive the advice, the more Edi is likely to kick back. Most people do not like receiving unwanted advice."

Asking permission can have several positive effects. It reinforces Edi's autonomy, it emphasizes the collaborative nature of the relationship, and it can also lower resistance. Generally, the more directive the advice, the more Edi is likely to kick back. Most people do not like receiving unwanted advice. Of course, there is also advice and information that is welcome and useful. Use sparingly and gauge how it is being received.

Offer choices

If you feel it is important to get some information across to Edi, try to offer choices. Again, this supports autonomy. If possible, offer several options simultaneously. This will reduce the opportunity for Edi to diligently go through your options crossing one off at a time or coming up with the 'Yeah, but ...' scenario. For example, 'We're going out for Tom's birthday lunch tomorrow. I know these sorts of things are difficult for you. A couple of options that may help are looking to see if there is an online menu or, if not, calling the restaurant ahead to get one. What do you think?'

Talk about what others do

When giving information, particularly if it contains implications for action, consider the value of talking about how this has affected, say, other sufferers. Quoting a 'higher being' often bears more weight than our own ideas. For example, 'Dr Thompson has already spoken to you about the extreme dangers involved in excessive exercise and low weight. I read a case study of his today that spoke of a young woman and the health challenges she was up against.'

Eliciting self-motivating statements

The aim of the motivational model is to gently nudge Edi to help them find their own motivation to change. This happens through encouragement and support and by recognizing that they are in charge of their recovery process and that they have the ability and creativity to come up with their own positive solutions and options.

You can support Edi by helping them come to realize the possible benefits of change. Instead of arguing about why change is necessary, it may be more conducive to try to elicit self-motivating statements. Keep a look out for 'gold nugget' statements, such as 'I'm so fed up of food controlling my thoughts', 'I so want to go back to university and have some sort of a life again'.

"If you do find a particular question has worked well, write it down and reflect on others that may nudge Edi in the right direction."

The following evocative questions can spark opportunities to elicit some self-motivating statements. You may even be able to think up some of your own that can be added to your personal toolkit. If you do find a particular question has worked well, write it down and reflect on others that may nudge Edi in the right direction. Here are some ideas to start you off...

- 'What's the downside of how you're feeling right now?'
- 'What are the advantages?'
- 'When you look at your friends and what they're doing right now, what are your thoughts on that?'
- 'What do you see yourself doing next year at this time?'

- 'Where do your beliefs and dreams for the future fit in with your current lifestyle?'

Asking for elaboration

By asking Edi to elaborate on what is being said, you show them they are really being listened to, as well as enhancing a greater understanding in terms of their perspective. It is an extension of reflective listening. Some examples are as follows:

- 'I found what you just said really interesting. What do you think are the triggers for these episodes?'
- 'I'm interested in … I'd like to know more, if that's okay with you.'

Visualization techniques

Therapists often use writing exercises as part of their visualization techniques. They might encourage Edi to look forward to a time when they do not have an eating disorder and look back to happier times before their eating disorder took a hold of their life. Looking forward also encourages Edi to think of the bigger picture rather than focusing on minute details, which is common in those suffering from an eating disorder (see page 37).

Looking forward

Encourage Edi to try to visualize their life in one year, two years, five years' time. What will it look like with the eating disorder still a strong presence in their lives? What will it look like without the eating disorder? How does it feel? What are they doing? Who are they with? This requires *very* careful listening after you've asked the question. The slightest hint of any change talk can then be handed back through careful reflective listening.

- 'Think ahead five years – what would your life be like if the eating disorder has left your life?'
- 'Suppose things don't change, where do you think you'll be five years from now?'

Looking back

Ask Edi to compare the present situation with the past situation. Often old family photographs or videos depicting happier times can be used – or reminiscing about past family holidays.

- 'Remember what your life was like five years ago?'
- 'What was happening?'
- 'How does this compare with what's happening now?'

Remember to go easy on yourself as you use the techniques in this chapter. Be your own scientist. Experiment and allow results to inform your next move. What works for one person in one situation will vary from another person or even the same individual in another setting. Develop and build your own toolbox and don't be afraid to make mistakes and then come back and try again. Hopefully, these examples can offer some new tools and ideas to work *with* Edi as opposed to, what may sometimes feel like, against them.

TIP

There are more examples of MI techniques being used in commonly occurring scenarios between carers and people with eating disorders on the New Maudsley website (see page 183).

8

NAVIGATING PROBLEMATIC BEHAVIOUR

As well as problematic eating behaviour, you may face a myriad of other challenging behaviours from Edi. As well as finding more effective ways of communicating with Edi, it also helps to have strategies to tackle the specific behavioural problems that can be associated with eating disorders. The following diagram illustrates a few examples. You may find yourself adding other challenging behaviours you have encountered. This chapter offers techniques that may help you address some of these difficult behaviours, including:

- Bingeing
- Vomiting
- Laxatives
- Over exercise
- Isolation

- Perfectionism
- Rituals and compulsions
- Cutting and self harm

THE ABC MODEL

Carers often find this model useful in addressing some of the problematic behaviours that accompany an eating disorder. The A stands for the antecedents – the triggers for the behaviour; B is the actual behaviours, and C the consequences of those behaviours. One of the main tools to help stop or reduce unacceptable behaviour is first to monitor how often it is happening. Keeping a notebook or diary is a useful way of jotting down, for example, binges or excessive exercise etc. You might find it useful to share it with Edi as a way of helping to nurture or encourage open and honest discussion around feelings or behaviours. The diary can be reviewed on a weekly basis, particularly if Edi finds it helpful and not too intrusive.

The ABC model can be effectively combined with MI. For example, rather than ignoring the signs of a binge, you might say, 'I noticed signs that you've had a binge. It could be helpful for us to have a chat and reflect on what happened. How would you feel about that?' The following scenario exemplifies the use of the ABC model.

CASE STUDY

Amy binged whilst her mum was at work. Her mum returns home to a kitchen and bathroom in complete upheaval. Amy is upset, her mum is upset and there are tears, angry words, and high emotions. A couple of hours later when all is calm again, they investigate the scenario objectively. Earlier that morning, Amy told her mum that she had planned to go shopping with her friend in the afternoon but at the last minute, her friend had cancelled. Amy felt let down, lonely, and unworthy … 'a crap person'. Using money that she found in her mum's bedroom, she went to the local shop, bought food, binged, and vomited.

Amy and her mum sit down and use the ABC model. They start to create a menu of options as to how they could address a similar situation, if it were to happen again.

Antecedent (trigger)	Behaviour	Consequence
Friend changes plans Feelings of disappointment trigger feelings of low self-worth and distress	Stealing money, bingeing, and vomiting	Initial relief from negative emotions followed by shame, disgust, and guilt Mess in kitchen and bathroom No food left in cupboards Criticism and hostility from Mum

MENU OF OPTIONS

Recognize triggers

Walk the dog

Make other plans

Contact a support person – friend, family member

Ask Mum to help limit access to large amounts of food for the short term

"If your responses are met with anger or derision, work with it. Thank Edi for explaining how they are feeling. Keep calm."

HOW TO BE AN EMOTIONAL COACH

When using the ABC model, it can be useful to work with the five basic steps of being an emotional coach: Attend, Label, Validate, Regulate and Learn.

1. **Attend:** Look and listen out for signs of rising or maladaptive emotions. *Attend* to those signs, e.g., 'I can sense that you're really upset about your plans being changed today.'

2. **Label:** Sometimes emotions may feel so overwhelming, Edi may have difficulty recognizing them, let alone naming them. Listen and watch carefully and gently coach and guide Edi as to what might be going on, e.g., 'Deep down you're hurt and disappointed and the overwhelming emotion that's coming out is one of anger.'

3. **Validate:** Use empathy to validate feelings. This may help Edi to acknowledge feelings and needs, e.g., 'I can understand why you're feeling like this. I don't like it either when I've planned to do something then it's changed at the last minute.' Don't brush these feelings off – listen very carefully and try to put yourself in Edi's shoes before responding.

4. **Regulate:** When responding, try to model more adaptive emotional responses without necessarily brushing off the negative emotions. We all feel strong emotions and it's a case of striking a balance without allowing the negative emotions to overcome us. If your responses are met with anger or derision, work with it. Thank Edi for explaining how they are feeling. Keep calm. If it becomes overwhelming for you, gently tell Edi this and take a break. Alternatively, would this be an appropriate moment for a hug?

5. **Learn:** Reflect on the situation afterwards. What did you learn from it? What worked? What didn't work? What would you do differently the next time, or the same?

SMART GOALS

If Edi is in one of the later stages of change, i.e., preparation, action, maintenance, it may be more appropriate to use more action-oriented approaches such as goal-setting. Setting small bite-sized goals may help provide clarity and a sense of direction and focus when considering the way forward. Goals should encompass a balanced approach; too easy and motivation may fall by the wayside, too difficult then self-esteem will plunge at the first hint of failure. Let's say, Amy (see case study on page 143) is open to setting herself some goals to include in her menu of options. First of all, it is important to set SMART goals – **S**pecific, **M**easurable, **A**chievable, **R**ealistic and **T**angible.

Specific: If Edi is willing to discuss goal setting, encourage her or him to think about what might be achieved in the short term. What are the hurdles, costs, constraints, and requirements, and how will they face any obstacles? Where appropriate, encourage them to establish a timeframe along with any support that they will need. A possible example:

Next time I feel distressed at any change of plans, I will write down my unhelpful thoughts, along with facts that support the thought and facts that provide evidence against the thoughts in order to try and achieve a more balanced perspective.

Measurable: Encourage Edi to establish concrete criteria for measuring progress toward the attainment of each goal set, e.g.

How will I know if I have made progress?
What will a small achievement or step in the right direction look like?

Achievable: Encourage Edi to think about the steps involved in reaching a goal, e.g.

I will share my thoughts with my therapist on this. She will help me examine whether my reaction is in proportion to what actually happened. I will come up with a list of options myself as soon as I recognize any triggers. I will go over these options and make sure that they are manageable and that I would feel comfortable with them.

Realistic: Remind Edi about the importance of being realistic. A goal must represent something that they feel is important enough for them to devote their time to and also that they are able to do. On the one hand, a goal should be challenging enough to be motivating and on the other, they do not want to set themselves up for failure.

I really do not want to continue to binge and vomit. I want to move forward in my life and leave the eating disorder behind me. I had been doing really well at reducing my bingeing and vomiting and I felt that this recent binge has set me back three steps. I find the shame and disgust unbearable. I will reward myself for any small achievements I make.

Tangible: A goal is tangible when you can experience it with one of the senses, i.e., taste, touch, smell, sight, or hearing. When a goal is tangible, one has a better chance of making it specific and measurable and thus achievable.

I will now write a clear and focused goal in my diary, which I will consult at the first sense of a trigger.

When I feel an unplanned occurrence is threatening my sense of self-worth, I will immediately spend some time writing down an alternative, more realistic and balanced perspective. I will then take the dog for a walk and call Mum or another friend for support if I think I need it.

"The problem with continuous reassurance is that although it may temporarily alleviate anxiety, it comes back even stronger within a short time."

THE REASSURANCE TRAP

Many carers find themselves being constantly drawn into the reassurance trap. It sometimes seems as if questions such as, 'Do I look fat?', 'Have I put on weight?', 'Have you given me a bigger plate than her?', 'Tell me again, how many grams of butter you put into this?' dominate every waking moment.

The problem with continuous reassurance is that although it may temporarily alleviate anxiety, it comes back even stronger within a short time. In reality, anxiety will normally level off naturally. In other words, it will have its own natural life span and so, with constant reassurance, Edi is not given the opportunity to show that they can tolerate distress. It is also unhelpful to have lengthy conversations that focus on food, weight, and shape.

There are a number of ways that you can work with the reassurance trap. One way is to externalize the eating disorder and by this, I mean give it a name – Ana, Gremlin, Boa Constrictor, Bob. Tell Edi that whilst you love and support them, you absolutely refuse to collude with and enable the eating disorder.

Another option is to explain that constant reassurance is unhelpful to Edi's recovery and that you will only reassure them once and that will be the 'reassurance quota' used up until the next day, when the same thing will happen. Look at this short piece of dialogue that gives one example of how to work with the reassurance trap:

Edi: *I can't believe how I look in this dress for the wedding on Saturday. I'm too fat for it. I don't have any time left to look for another. I just feel so overweight. How do you think I look?*

Mark: *We spoke about this last night. I said you looked fantastic in it, but Annie Anorexia won't allow you to consider or accept that.* (**Complex reflection**)

Edi: *That is not true. I just need you to let me know how it really is.*

Mark: *We discussed with the nurse at the workshop how reassurance wasn't helpful and that it just feeds that monster screaming in your ear. I know you're getting really distressed and I do want to be there for you when the going gets tough. On the other hand, I don't want to get into lengthy discussions about this kinda stuff as I don't think it's helpful.* (**Mark sets boundaries, reiterates both his support as well as the reason why he won't get caught up in the reassurance trap**)

Edi: *That's bullshit. Look, Mark, I just need your reassurance. I'll ask Mum if you won't give it.*

Mark: *How about we meet in the middle? We can talk about the dress and how it looks for the next five minutes. We'll then park all that talk and get on with something else. I really don't think it's helpful as it I feel it's only feeding 'Annie'. Actually,*

I'd much prefer talking about the day itself, about how it'll be great to see Sandi and all the rest of the gang. (**Mark offers a compromise, again emphasizing his wish not to collude with the eating disorder. Instead, he opens up the conversation to the bigger picture, introducing non-eating disorder talk.**)

Edi: *I'm looking forward to the day too.*

Mark: *I know you are. It is hard for you and you've been working so well fighting back against this illness. Let's help send that voice to its corner. I think you look amazing in the dress although I am more interested in how you feel.* (**Mark offers empathy and praise as well as turning the conversation away from weight and shape talk to what's going on in terms of 'feelings'**)

Edi: *Guess it's the usual anxiety taking over.*

Mark: *If you're OK with me putting a cap on the reassurance, I can support you in tackling the anxiety. How do you feel about working with that journal we started and you coming up with different ways to deal with 'Annie' when she begins to shout too loud?*

In her skills training manual, Janet Treasure talks about the APT (Awareness, Planning, and Trying) cornerstones of working to change habits.[36] In the above scenario, for example, Mark raises Awareness of Jane's need for reassurance as well as the dangers of him giving constant reassurance. If Jane is open to exploring this further, she could begin to document examples of every time she feels a strong need for reassurance to alleviate her anxiety. She could then use a Planning stage, perhaps in a journal, to come up with different ways to address her anxiety and of how she could tackle it the next time around. Trying out these ideas next time will eventually enable her to learn what works, what she can learn from previous times or mistakes, since everybody makes them.

DARN-CATS (see page 105) can also be used to address any problematic behaviour. Whilst motivation is in the wavering stage, DARN (Desire, Ability, Reasons, and Need) will be required to elicit and work with preparatory change talk with the goal of guiding any discussions or conversations toward increasingly action-orientated *change* talk, at which point you can begin to work with CATS (Commitment, Activation Talk, Taking Steps). Once this has been established or you recognize a stronger disposition toward change talk, you may be able to move on to SMART goals.

REMEMBER

This will not be a linear process. Keep in mind, the motivational dance as opposed to struggle. Gauge the responses, move back a few steps, or walk away for a while if needs be.

"It is important to remember that when Edi vocalizes future plans, this holds more strength than advice from others and is more likely to actually happen."

Recognize those golden moments when Edi wavers between preparatory change talk and retaining the status quo. These may include questions about the consequences of the eating disorder and how these impact on future plans and goals. Work with this talk. Reflect on what Edi is saying. If you feel resistance, move back a bit. If change talk continues, move toward activation talk. Elicit from *them* how they see this happening, the potential obstacles and how they will address these, small steps that they can take toward goals, and how you can support them. It is important to remember that when Edi vocalizes future plans, this holds more strength than advice from others and is more likely to actually happen.

9

TAKING CARE OF YOURSELF

When it comes to your own self-care, as a carer, the New Maudsley Approach uses the analogy of an oxygen mask when you are flying. In the event of an emergency, you are instructed on how to fit your oxygen mask and told to put your own mask on first before attending to others. It is the same scenario when supporting somebody with an eating disorder, whether it be your child, your partner, your sister, brother, or friend. To be the best support to Edi, you must make sure you put your own mask on first.

> "Eating disorders are exhausting and destructive. It is important to nurture adaptive coping mechanisms that assist in buoying up your own sense of wellbeing."

Not only is it important for you to look after your own psychological and physical wellbeing, but it also sends an important message to Edi. In looking after your needs, you are role-modelling your determination not to allow the eating disorder to destroy every last aspect of family, relationships, social life, routine, and day-to-day life.

> "In looking after your needs, you are role-modelling your determination not to allow the eating disorder to destroy every aspect of life."

Consequently, parents need to take some time out to nurture their own relationship, siblings need some time out with or without other family members, partners need to reach out and speak to other people. Eating disorders are exhausting and destructive. It is important to nurture adaptive coping mechanisms that assist in buoying up your own sense of wellbeing.

In her training manual, Jenny Langley has devised a framework intended to encourage reflection on your own needs and how you might address these.[37]

It involves comparing your current happiness with your happiness before the eating disorder came into your life, considering the reason for this change and creating steps to improve this happiness level. Here's an example:

My happiness with:	My physical health
Current happiness (0–10)	5
Happiness before ED (0–10)	10
Reason for the change	*Exhausted, stressed*
Steps I can take to make improvements	*Eat better, take up yoga again, have more 'me' time*
Rank out of 10, any obstacles to change	*9*
How I will address obstacles	*Devise action plan sheet for myself. Join yoga class.* *Use 'If/Then' table on page 158.*

ACTIVITY:
Improving Self-care

Create a table following the above as a guide for different aspects of your life, including your: physical health, social life, job, hobbies, financial issues and emotional health. Consider also your relationships, including your relationship with: your partner/spouse, Edi, other children, close friends, extended family, parent/siblings etc.

On completion of this exercise, reflect on how you will address the obstacles to make your action plan a greater reality. Remember to use SMART goals (see page 146).

In addition to using SMART goals, you may find the following 'If/Then' contingency table a useful tool to help you reflect on a way forward.

IF	THEN
I'm feeling exhausted, depressed, stressed …	• Make an appointment with my doctor. • Contemplate therapy.
I've cut ties with all my friends …	• Make a point of calling old friends up for a chat, schedule a coffee, glass of wine.
I'm missing my job, due to having given it up to look after Edi …	• Touch base with old colleagues. • Perhaps look into working on a part-time basis.

IF	THEN
My relationship with my partner is suffering because we spend no time with each other …	<ul><li>Schedule a night away, dinner etc.</li><li>Make a point to have a non-eating disorder conversation for at least half the evening.</li></ul>
My relationship with my other children is suffering …	<ul><li>Plan activities with other children that don't necessarily involve Edi.</li><li>Ask friends to look after Edi for an afternoon to allow non-eating disorder activities to happen.</li><li>Be mindful of their needs – empathize and communicate.</li></ul>

10

NEXT STEPS

Most carers, including those whose loved ones have been recovered for several years, will tell you that the nature of eating disorders is three steps forward, two steps back. Sometimes, it may even feel like three steps forward, four steps back! The maintenance period can come with its own stresses. Yes, we are absolutely delighted that the problematic behaviours are decreasing or have even disappeared; however, we are still concerned with the 'What Ifs'. For example:

- What happens if they do not get into their university of choice?
- What happens if they are made redundant from their job?
- What happens if they suffer a bereavement?
- What happens if they have a relationship breakdown?

The list is endless.

If Edi moves away to university or for work, it may be difficult for you to let go. If Edi is in the maintenance phase and you find yourself still stressed out on a regular basis, particularly with regards to any potential pitfalls that can arise. Trust issues, for example, will have likely been a challenge for some time, due to the very nature of an eating disorder and any deceit or lies over what is being eaten. Consequently, it may be difficult for you to truly believe that Edi is capable of looking after his or her wellbeing independently.

Some carers I have worked with have also reported a sense of loss after Edi moves on with his or her life. Supporting someone with an eating disorder is an all-encompassing role. It may have dominated your life for so long that it becomes difficult to adapt, recover and build one's own life again. Work may have been given up long ago to care for Edi. Social networks may have become neglected. It may prove daunting to pick up the strings of normal life again. Carers themselves may feel the need to enter therapy. If necessary, talk to your doctor regarding your own needs. There are also several organizations and care groups around the country for carers of people with eating disorders. Links are posted at the end of this book.

Whilst the contingency planning 'If/Then' table at the end of Chapter 9 addresses your needs as a carer, the following table addresses life situations that could create stress and lead to setbacks in Edi. You may want to add some of your own. If Edi is open to discussing contingency plans, perhaps they can also think of their own set of options.

IF	THEN
Bereavement	• Bereavement counselling. • Remind Edi of the positive coping strategies they have developed: 'You have proved you can overcome emotional difficulties'. • Listen to their thoughts and feelings: 'I am here if you would like to talk some more'. • Remind Edi that it is okay to feel sad.
Relationships breakdown	• Listen, love, empathize. • Let Edi know you are there for them. • Encourage Edi to keep up or renew links with friends, hobbies, travel plans etc. • Distract with other activities they enjoy.
Low self-esteem or confidence levels	• Talk and listen. • Text/write/email if that is easier for them to start with. • Affirm their qualities, point out their skills, strengths, and unique features.

IF	THEN
Low self-esteem or confidence levels continued	• Point out how they have addressed challenging situations and their coping strategies in the past. • Look at the bigger picture of future life opportunities. • Pull in support network. • Consider counselling if it is becoming a big issue.
Periods returning	• Acknowledge any inner turmoil relating to this. • Look at the positives: 'return to health, opportunity to have a family'. • Empathize (PMT, period pain, inconvenience etc.) • Offer distractions.
Weight falling	• Remind them of consequences (adverse effects on the brain, anxiety, treatment etc.). • Listen – are they feeling out of control, or is there something else bothering them? • Praise that they have beaten an eating disorder before. • How did they deal with difficulties before and were those difficulties overcome? • What support did they need? • Be prepared to act, if weight gets dangerously low.

IF	THEN
Weight rising	• Recognize emotions likely to be in turmoil and this might lead to irrational behaviour. • Acknowledge fear. • Talk about it. If bingeing, is the ABC model (see page 142) appropriate? • Watch out for signs of bingeing and/or purging. • Help them find the right balance and accept that it will take some time.
Exam pressure/Job problems	• Acknowledge difficulties. • Help look at all options. • Support through tough times. • Remind them life is not all about exams/job – help them see the big picture. • Remind them of strategies they have used in previous challenging circumstances. • Teach self-compassion and the futility of striving for perfection.

CONCLUSION

I hope that this book has offered some practical tools and techniques for those of you supporting someone with an eating disorder. You will undoubtedly be living on a rollercoaster of extreme emotions and I cannot stress enough the importance of looking after your own emotional needs.

It is crucial that you remember that you are not expected to become an expert in MI, or Edi's therapist. This book is intended to be used as a reference, a support tool. You are the expert. If something is or is not working, keep a note of it. Work with this knowledge and experiment with different techniques and responses. Above all, be kind and compassionate to yourself.

Supporting someone through an eating disorder is no easy task. By being compassionate to yourself, accepting when communication does and does not go the right way, you will be sending an important message out to Edi. It is okay to make mistakes and life does not always go to plan. I would like to close the book with a quote from a recovered sufferer reflecting on the role of the carer.

"Carers must not feel that their support falls on deaf ears. The knowledge may not be used until the sufferer is ready to accept recovery, but a seed has been sown for the future. Personally, I heard every word but just wasn't ready to use it until the time was right. Please don't give up on us."

Finally, I would like to wish each and every one of you all the very best for a happy and healthy future ahead. You are doing a brilliant job.

APPENDIX

ACCOMMODATION AND ENABLING SCALE FOR EATING DISORDERS

The following items contain a number of statements that commonly apply to the family members who live with relatives or friends with an eating disorder. Read each one and decide how often it has applied to you and your family members over the *past one month*. It is important to note that there are no right or wrong answers. Your first reaction will usually provide the best answer.

This is adapted from *Development and validation of the accommodation and enabling scale for eating disorders (AESED) for caregivers in eating disorders.*[38]

DURING THE PAST MONTH, HOW OFTEN HAVE YOU THOUGHT ABOUT THE FOLLOWING:

Answer: *0 = never, 1 = rarely, 2 = sometimes, 3 = often, 4 = every day*

	Does Edi control:					
1.	The choices of food that you buy?	0	1	2	3	4
2.	What other family members do, and for how long, in the kitchen?	0	1	2	3	4
3.	Cooking practice and ingredients you use?	0	1	2	3	4
4.	What other family members eat?	0	1	2	3	4
	Does Edi engage any family member in repeated conversations:					
5.	Asking for reassurance about whether she/he will get fat?	0	1	2	3	4
6.	About whether it is safe or acceptable to eat certain food?	0	1	2	3	4
7.	Asking for reassurance about whether she/he looks fat in certain clothes?	0	1	2	3	4
8.	About ingredients and amounts, possible substitutes for ingredients?	0	1	2	3	4
9.	About negative thoughts and feelings?	0	1	2	3	4
10.	About self-harm?	0	1	2	3	4
	Do any family members have to accommodate to the following:					
11.	What crockery is used?	0	1	2	3	4
12.	How crockery is cleaned?	0	1	2	3	4
13.	What time food is eaten?	0	1	2	3	4
14.	What place food is eaten?	0	1	2	3	4

15.	How the kitchen is cleaned?	0	1	2	3	4
16.	How food is stored?	0	1	2	3	4
17.	The exercise routine of the relative with an ED?	0	1	2	3	4
18.	Your friend/relative checking their body shape or weight?	0	1	2	3	4
19.	How the house is cleaned and tidied?	0	1	2	3	4

Do you choose to ignore aspects of Edi's eating disorder that impinge on your family's life in an effort to reconcile or make it tolerable for the rest of the family, such as if:

20.	Food disappears?	0	1	2	3	4
21.	Money is taken?	0	1	2	3	4
22.	The kitchen is left a mess?	0	1	2	3	4
23.	The bathroom is left a mess?	0	1	2	3	4

24. In general, to what extent would you say that Edi controls family life and activities?

None at All					About Half				Completely	
0	1	2	3	4	5	6	7	8	9	10

DURING THE PAST MONTH, HOW OFTEN HAS THE FOLLOWING OCCURRED:

Answer: 0 = never, 1 = 1-3 times/month, 2 = 1-2 times/week, 3 = 3-6 times/week, 4 = daily

25.	How often did you participate in behaviours related to Edi's compulsions?	0	1	2	3	4
26.	How often did you assist your relative in avoiding things that might make Edi more anxious?	0	1	2	3	4

DURING THE PAST MONTH, CONSIDER:

Answer: *0 = no, 1 = mild, 2 = moderate, 3 = severe, 4 = extreme*

27.	Have you avoided doing things, going to places, or being with people because of Edi's disorder?	0	1	2	3	4
28.	Have you modified your family routine because of Edi's symptoms?	0	1	2	3	4
29.	Have you modified your work schedule because of Edi's needs?	0	1	2	3	4
30.	Have you modified your leisure activities because of Edi's needs?	0	1	2	3	4
31.	Has helping Edi in the before mentioned ways caused you distress?	0	1	2	3	4
32.	Has Edi become distressed/anxious when you have not provided assistance?	0	1	2	3	4
33.	Has Edi become angry/abusive when you have not provided assistance?	0	1	2	3	4

ACKNOWLEDGEMENTS

I would like to thank Professor Janet Treasure and colleagues and all the researchers and coaches who have worked on various iterations of the carer skills training interventions at King's College, London. Their continued dedication and motivation to develop interventions for both sufferers and carers continues to inspire. I would also like to thank all the sufferers and carers who have participated in the continuing phases of the research projects. Together they make a formidable team!

ENDNOTES

1. Treasure, J., U. Schmidt, and P. Macdonald, *The Clinician's Guide to Collaborative Caring in Eating Disorders*. 2010, London: Routledge.

2. Treasure, J., G. Smith, and A. Crane, *Skills-based caring for a loved one with an eating disorder: The New Maudsley Method. (2nd Ed.)*. 2nd ed. 2017, London: Routledge.

3. Treasure, J., G. Smith, and A. Crane, *Skills-based caring for a loved one with an eating disorder: The New Maudsley Method. (2nd Ed.)*. 2nd ed. 2017, London: Routledge.

4. Diagnostic and Statistical Manual of Mental Disorders (DSM-IV)

5. Morgan, J., Reid, F., Lacey, J., *The SCOFF questionnaire: assessment of a new screening tool for eating disorders*. British Medical Journal, 1999. **319**(7223): p. 1467-1468.

6. NICE. Eating Disorders: Recognition and Treatment. NICE guideline [ng69]. Published 23 May 2017. www.nice.org.uk/guidance/ng69

7. Morgan, J., Reid, F., Lacey, J., *The SCOFF questionnaire: assessment of a new screening tool for eating disorders. .* British Medical Journal, 1999. **319**(7223): p. 1467-1468.

8. Langley, J., G. Todd, and J. Treasure, *Caring for a loved one with an eating disorder. The New Maudsley skills-based training manual.* 2019, London: Routledge.

9. Zabala, M., P. Macdonald, and J. Treasure, *Appraisal of caregiving burden, expressed emotion and psychological distress in families of people with eating disorders: A systematic review.* European Eating Disorders Review, 2009. **17**(5): p. 338-349.

10. ibid

11. Treasure, J., G. Smith, and A. Crane, *Skills-based caring for a loved one with an eating disorder: The New Maudsley Method. (2nd Ed.).* 2nd ed. 2017, London: Routledge

12. Langley, J., G. Todd, and J. Treasure, *Caring for a loved one with an eating disorder. The New Maudsley skills-based training manual.* 2019, London: Routledge.

13. Linville, D., et al., *Reciprocal influence of couple dynamics and eating disorders.* Journal of Marital and Family Therapy, 2015. **42**(2): p. 326-340.

14. Pinheiro, A.P., et al., *Sexual functioning in women with eating disorders.* International Journal of Eating Disorders, 2010. **43**: p. 123-129.

15. Treasure, J., G. Smith, and A. Crane, *Skills-based caring for a loved one with an eating disorder: The New Maudsley Method. (2nd Ed.).* 2nd ed. 2017, London: Routledge.

16. Ibid

17. Gilbert, P., *The Compassionate Mind.* 2009, London: Constable.

18. Treasure, J., et al., *Interpersonal maintaining factors in eating disorders: Skill sharing interventions for carers.* International Journal of Child and Adolescent Health, 2008. **1**(4): p. 331-338.

19. Treasure, J., U. Schmidt, and P. Macdonald, *The Clinician's Guide to Collaborative Caring in Eating Disorders.* 2010, London: Routledge.

20. Butzlaff, R.L. and J.M. Hooley, *Expressed emotion and psychiatric relapse: A meta-analysis.* Arch Gen Psychiatry, 1998. **55**: p. 547-552.

21. Sepulveda, A.R., O. Kyriacou, and J. Treasure, *Development and validation of the accommodation and enabling scale for eating disorders (AESED) for caregivers in eating disorders.* BMC Health Serv Res, 2009. **9**: p. 171. doi: 10.1186/2050-2974-1-13.

22. Treasure, J., G. Smith, and A. Crane, *Skills-based caring for a loved one with an eating disorder: The New Maudsley Method. (2nd Ed.).* 2nd ed. 2017, London: Routledge.

23. Prochaska, J. and C. DiClemente, *The Transtheoretical Approach: Crossing the Traditional Boundaries of Therapy.* 1984, Homewood, IL: Dow Jones Irwen.

24. Ibid

25. Treasure, J., *Anorexia nervosa: A survival guide for families, friends and sufferers.* 2005, Routledge: London. p. 139-145

26. Schmidt, U. and J. Treasure, *Anorexia nervosa: Valued and visible. A cognitive-interpersonal maintenance model and its implications for research and practice.* British Journal of Clinical Psychology, 2006. **45**: p. 343-366.

27. Ibid

28. Miller, W.R. and S. Rollnick, *Motivational Interviewing: Helping People Change (Third Edition).* 2013, New York: The Guildford Press.

29. Ibid

30. Ibid

31. Rollnick, S., W.R. Miller, and C.C. Butler, *Motivational Interviewing in Health Care.* 2008, New York: The Guildford Press.

32. Miller, W.R. and S. Rollnick, *Motivational Interviewing: Helping People Change (Third Edition)*. 2013, New York: The Guildford Press.

33. Ibid

34. Macdonald, P., et al., *Disseminating skills to carers of people with eating disorders: An examination of treatment fidelity in lay and professional carer coaches.* Health Psychology and Behavioral Medicine, 2014. **2**(1): p. 555-564.

35. Miller, W.R. and S. Rollnick, *Motivational Interviewing: Helping People Change (Third Edition)*. 2013, New York: The Guildford Press.

36. Treasure, J., G. Smith, and A. Crane, *Skills-based caring for a loved one with an eating disorder: The New Maudsley Method. (2nd Ed.).* 2nd ed. 2017, London: Routledge.

37. Langley, J., G. Todd, and J. Treasure, *Caring for a loved one with an eating disorder. The New Maudsley skills-based training manual.* 2019, London: Routledge.

38. Sepulveda, A.R., O. Kyriacou, and J. Treasure, *Development and validation of the accommodation and enabling scale for eating disorders (AESED) for caregivers in eating disorders.* BMC Health Serv Res, 2009. **9**: p. 171. doi: 10.1186/2050-2974-1-13.

USEFUL RESOURCES

GLOBAL

- Boy Anorexia: resources aimed specifically at families supporting boys through an eating disorder. www.boyanorexia.com

- Global Foundation for Eating Disorders (GFED): www.gfed.org

- International Eating Disorder Family Support (IEDFS) facebook group: www.facebook.com/groups/International. Eating.Disorder.Family.Support.IEDFS

- International Eating Disorder Referral Organization: provides information and treatment resources for all forms of eating disorders. www.edreferral.com

- Lock, J and Le Grange, D, *Help your Teenager Beat an Eating Disorder* (Guildford Press, 2015). This book has a comprehensive list of international clinics in their resources at the back.

- Project Heal (found in the US, Canada and Australia): www.theprojectheal.org

UK

- Anorexia Bulimia Care: if you are over 18 they offer a befriending scheme. www.anorexiabulimiacare.org.uk

- BEAT: provides online and phone support for patients and carers. www.beateatingdisorders.org.uk

- First Steps ED: a fantastic charity that focuses massively on early intervention, giving you a space to come and speak up. firststepsed.co.uk

- Freedfromed.co.uk: this is a network of NHS organizations offering early intervention support.

- Eating Disorder Association Northern Ireland: www.eatingdisordersni.co.uk

- The Laurence Trust: www.thelaurencetrust.co.uk

- New Maudsley Approach: A resource for professionals and carers of people with eating disorders, focusing on the work of Professor Janet Treasure and her team at King's College, London. Also offers online training for carers and professionals in the New Maudsley Approach. www.thenewmaudsleyapproach.co.uk

- New Maudsley Carers: support and information for carers that provides resources, worksheets, and videos using the New Maudsley approach. www.newmaudsleycarers-kent.co.uk

- NHS: www.nhs.uk/conditions/eating-disorders

- Support ED: offers psychoeducational help, guidance and support to carers in Scotland. www.supportedscotland.org

- Veronica Kamerling: therapist supporting families with mental health issues. www.eatingdisordersandcarers.co.uk

- YoungMinds: young people's mental health charity. youngminds.org.uk; parent helpline 0808 8025544

US

- Alliance for Eating Disorders:
  www.allianceforeatingdisorders.com

- American Psychological Association: provides information
  and links for people with eating disorders.
  www.apa.org/topics/eating-disorders

- Eating Disorder Hope: www.eatingdisorderhope.com/
  treatment-for-eating-disorders/international

- FEAST: provides support, advice, and guidance for parents
  in accessing appropriate treatment and equipping families
  with information. www.feast-ed.org

- National Association of Anorexia Nervosa and Associated
  Disorders (ANAD): anad.org

- National Eating Disorders Association (NEDA): this
  organization has some brilliant blogs as well as a
  crisis text messenger service and helpline.
  www.nationaleatingdisorders.org

AUSTRALIA

- The Butterfly Foundation: butterfly.org.au

SPECIFIC LINKS

Additional examples of Motivational Interviewing techniques on the New Maudsley website: thenewmaudsleyapproach.co.uk/pdfs/MI-roleplay-scenarios. pdf

Assessing Medical Risk: thenewmaudsleyapproach.co.uk/media/Medical_risk.pdf

Measure used to determine the presence of an eating disorder: www.verywellmind.com/the-scoff-questionnaire-1138316

MARSIPAN checklist: www.rcpsych.ac.uk/docs/default-source/members/faculties/ eating-disorders/marsipan/eating-disorders-cr189-checklist. pdf?sfvrsn=d6ce3bb1_4

Useful aid in preparing for an initial doctor's consultation: www.beateatingdisorders.org.uk/uploads/documents/2017/ 10/gp-leaflet-website.pdf

MIND's leaflet entitled *Find the Words – Talking to Your GP About Mental Health*: www.mind.org.uk/findthewords

A document produced by South London and Maudsley that helps balance privacy and confidentiality with the best interest of service users.

m.slam.nhs.uk/media/13524/carers-and-confidentiality.pdf

FURTHER READING

Alexander, J., LeGrange, D., (2010). *My Kid Is Back: Empowering Parents to Beat Anorexia Nervosa.* London: Routledge.

Miller, W. R., Rollnick, S. (2002). *Motivational Interviewing: Preparing People for Change*, 2nd Edition. New York: Guildford.

Treasure, J., (1997). *Anorexia nervosa: a survival guide for families, friends and sufferers.* London: Routledge.

Treasure, J., Schmidt, U., (1997). *Getting better bit(e) by bit(e): a survival kit for sufferers of bulimia nervosa and binge eating disorders.* London: Routledge.

Treasure, J., Smith, G., Crane, A. (2016). *Skills-based learning for caring for a loved one with an eating disorder: The New Maudsley Method*, 2nd Edition. London: Routledge.

ABOUT US

Welbeck Balance publishes books dedicated to changing lives. Our mission is to deliver life enhancing books to help improve your wellbeing so that you can live your life with greater clarity and meaning, wherever you are on life's journey. Our Trigger books are specifically devoted to opening up conversations about mental health and wellbeing.

Welbeck Balance and Trigger are part of the Welbeck Publishing Group – a globally recognized independent publisher based in London. Welbeck are renowned for our innovative ideas, production values and developing long-lasting content. Our books have been translated into over 30 languages in more than 60 countries around the world.

If you love books, then join the club and sign up to our newsletter for exclusive offers, extracts, author interviews and more information.

To find out more and sign up, visit: www.welbeckpublishing.com

𝕏 welbeckpublish
⊙ welbeckpublish
f welbeckuk

Find out more about Trigger: www.triggerhub.org

𝕏 Triggercalm
f Triggercalm
⊙ Triggercalm

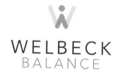

WELBECK
BALANCE